Also available from Quay Books, MA Healthcare Limited:

Trends in Wound Care, volume I edited by Richard J White

Trends in Wound Care, volume II edited by Richard J White

A–Z Dictionary of Wound Care by Fiona Collins, Sylvie Hampton and Richard White

Pressure Ulcers: Recent Advances in Tissue Viability edited by Michael Clark

Fundamental Aspects of Tissue Viability Nursing by Cheryl Dunford and Bridgit Günnewicht

Trends in Wound Care
volume III

edited by
Richard J White

Quay Books
MA Healthcare Limited

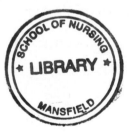

Quay Books Division, MA Healthcare Limited, Jesses Farm, Snow Hill, Dinton, Salisbury, Wiltshire, SP3 5HN

British Library Cataloguing-in-Publication Data
A catalogue record is available for this book

Printed by Cromwell Press, Trowbridge

Contents

List of contributors

Subhash Anand is Professor of Technical Textiles, Centre for Materials Research and Innovation, Bolton Institute, Bolton

Sue Bale is Director of Nursing at the Gwent Health Care NHS Trust, Cwmbran

Pauline Beldon is Tissue Viability Nurse Consultant, Epsom and St Helier University Hospitals NHS Trust, Epsom

Michael Clark is Senior Research Fellow, Wound Healing Research Unit, University of Wales College of Medicine, Cardiff

Keith F Cutting is Principle Lecturer at Buckingham Chilterns University College, Chalfont St Giles and Clinical Research Consultant, Chorleywood

Catherine Dean is Senior Lecturer, Department of Psychology and Life Sciences, Bolton Institute, Bolton

Keith G Harding is Head of Department of Surgery and Professor of Rehabilitation Medicine (wound healing) at University of Wales College of Medicine, Cardiff

Alan BG Lansdown is Senior Research Fellow, Medical Writer, Honorary Senior Lecturer in Chemical Pathology, Imperial College, London

Keith Moore is a freelance Scientist, WoundSci, Usk

Robert Nettleton is Principal Lecturer, Department of Health, Social and Community Studies, Bolton Institute, Bolton

Venkatraman Praburaj is Researcher, Centre for Materials Research and Innovation, Bolton Institute, Bolton

Kathryn Vowden is Nurse Consultant, acute and chronic wounds, Bradford Royal Infirmary, Bradford

Peter Vowden is Consultant Vascular Surgeon, Department of Vascular Surgery, Bradford Royal Infirmary, Bradford

Richard J White is a Clinical Research Consultant and Senior Research Fellow, Department of Tissue Viability, Aberdeen Royal Infirmary

Foreword

This is the third volume of *Trends in Wound Care* edited by Dr Richard White. It provides, yet again, a miscellany of interesting, challenging and practically relevant series of subjects that should be of interest to all clinicians interested in this subject. The first section addresses a number of practical aspects of wound healing, whereas the second section deals with the challenge of evidence and theory in wound care.

The first section deals with exudate, maceration and exudate composition. These three chapters address both the scientific base of this aspect of wound care, in addition to providing practical advice for clinicians. The chapters are well illustrated and the use of key points is helpful. The chapter on skin grafts provides a very comprehensive and readable review of this important and often forgotten wound type seen in clinical practice. The final chapter in this section is from my own group and may provide a solution to dealing with patients who are unable to use normal forms of compression. It is also likely to raise more questions for many clinicians who may not accept the research findings, but who should be encouraged to undertake their own research in this area.

The second section provides a review of the literature dealing with the use of silver in wound healing. It identifies the facts and issues surrounding this subject and should encourage clinicians to ask what, when and how they should choose silver containing products in their own practice. The challenge of diagnosing and managing infection in clinical practice is something we are all troubled by. The chapter on infection provides new information and new thinking on this subject. The last three chapters deal with issues as diverse as health-related quality of life, the scientific basis for compromised healing and challenges associated with the implementation of guidelines, all subjects which provoke debate and discussion in the field of wound healing. They provide a thorough review of these subjects in a practically relevant way and should encourage all readers to think more.

The third volume of *Trends in Wound Care* is, in my opinion, the best yet and helps to challenge clinicians working in this area so that they may adopt a more professional approach to this area of clinical practice.

Keith Harding
Head of University Department of Surgery
Professor of Rehabilitation Medicine (wound healing)
May 2004

Introduction

In this, the third volume of the series, I have attempted to refine and focus the coverage to specific key areas of topical interest. The overall theme is of improved patient outcomes and reduced morbidity associated with wounds. For chronic wounds in particular, a focus on 'compromised healing', exudate, infection criteria, maceration and quality of life is consistent with this theme. For acute wounds, a review of skin grafting is timely, especially as donor site management is also updated. The assembled authors are expert in their respective fields. The resulting chapters, each updated in recent months, reflect the most up-to-date research, opinion and clinical practice in this rapidly changing field of patient care.

Richard J White
Whitstone, June 2004

Acknowledgements

The editor and authors are indebted to Binkie Mais for her invaluable input into the organisation and preparation of this book. The editor is grateful to Edward Rusling for his constant support in the publication of this series.

Section one:
Practical aspects of wound care

1

The role of exudate in the healing process: understanding exudate management

Kathryn Vowden, Peter Vowden

Studies suggest that wound fluid from acute wounds may have a beneficial effect on wound healing, whereas that of chronic wounds may inhibit healing. Changes in the volume and nature of exudate provide information on the underlying state of the wound and may give an indication of an increasing bacterial load and the presence of infection, and if a wound is likely to proceed to healing. Careful monitoring of the exudate can provide information for the application of systemic and local therapies. Individual wound care products have specific functions which relate to the volume, viscosity and nature of the exudate and these should guide skin care and dressing selection.

Phenomenological studies have indicated that, to the patient, pain, odour and exudate are the three most important elements of a chronic wound and that they impact directly on a patient's quality of life (Hansson, 1997; Ovens and Fairhurst, 2002). Of these exudate is often the most important, since by controlling exudate the effect of the other two elements is often reduced.

The wound healing process

Wound healing is a complex process involving the interaction of many cell types, matrix components and biological factors, including growth factors, proteinases and cytokines within a fluid environment (Baker and Leaper, 2000). Like many aspects of wound care, successful exudate management is about achieving a balance within this fluid environment (Bishop *et al*, 2003).

Winter's theory of moist wound healing (1962) indicates the benefit of moisture in the healing of an acute wound, but excessive moisture can be deleterious, leading to skin maceration and wound complications. To date, no reliable functional definition exists as to what constitutes too little or too much wound surface moisture (Bolton *et al*, 2000). Little is known about the correct moisture balance in a chronic wound, although it is reasonable to assume that the same basic principles should apply for chronic and acute wounds.

It does appear that excessive fluid is not by itself the cause of delayed wound healing (Vogt *et al*, 1995) but that it is the nature of the fluid that is of primary importance (Bishop *et al*, 2003). The goal of effective wound management is to remove excess moisture, debris and 'chemicals' from the

3

wound surface while maintaining the ideal moisture balance to allow cell migration and ultimately wound healing. In some wounds this will parallel a process of wound debridement (Vowden and Vowden, 2002). For some chronic wounds, such as malignant ulcers, healing can be an unrealistic goal. In such circumstances symptom management, and in particular dressing performance and exudate control, are essential to maintain the patient's quality of life (Grocott, 1997; 2000).

Starling's equation (Partsch, 2003) indicates that a balance exists between the intravascular and extravascular fluid space. The fluid-handling power of the dermis is, in part, related to the fluid-binding capacity of the extracellular matrix (ECM). In the presence of a wound this balance is disrupted as the tissue containment fields are breached and the ECM often reduced (Bishop *et al*, 2003). This produces a pressure gradient which favours the production of exudate (*Figure 1.1*). It has been suggested that occlusive dressings, such as hydrocolloids, manage exudate not by absorption but by restoring the pressure gradient at the wound bed (Thomas, 1997a).

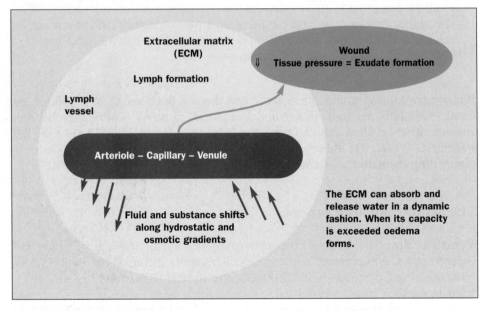

Figure 1.1: Diagrammatic representation of the generation of exudate

The imbalance that results from wounding may be further disturbed by underlying medical conditions, such as chronic venous hypertension, lymphatic or heart failure, by an inflammatory process such as rheumatoid arthritis, or by infection. *Table 1.1* outlines the factors that will affect Starling's equation and therefore alter tissue fluid level and oedema production, which in turn will change exudate volume and constituents and therefore the viscosity of the exudate. This will change the effect of the exudate on both the wound bed and the surrounding skin.

Table 1.1: Starling's equation (adapted from Partsch, 2003)

$$F = c(Pc - Pt) - (\pi c - \pi t)$$

F represents net filtration force (the origin of lymph); c is the filtration coefficient; **Pc** is the tissue pressure; πc is the capillary oncotic pressure; πt is tissue oncotic pressure

Physiology	Possible cause	Effect
$\neq$ Capillary permeability (c)	Cellulitis, arthritis, cyclic oedema hormonal	Inflammatory oedema; 'idiopathic oedema'
$\neq$ Venous (capillary) pressure (Pc)	Heart failure, venous insufficiency, dependency syndrome	Cardiac, venous oedema, dependent oedema
$\neq$ Oncotic tissue pressure (pt)	Failure of lymphatic drainage	Lymphoedema
$\emptyset$ Oncotic capillary pressure (pc)	Hypoalbuminaemia, nephritic syndrome, hepatic failure	Hypoproteinaemic oedema

As the equation moves to favour the formation of oedema, so exudate production will increase.

The role of wound exudate

A consistent factor in all chronic wounds is a prolonged inflammatory response (Moore, 1999), with cell types typical of inflammation being present in wound exudate (Buchan *et al*, 1980). Inflammation leads to an increase in vasodilatation and vessel permeability. In this way there is continual additional extracellular fluid formation, and this usually results in an increased and prolonged production of wound fluid and exudate.

Exudate levels are generally categorized as light, moderate or heavy (Watret, 1997). However, as White (2001) states, these categories are subjective and frequently inadequate to classify accurately or manage chronic wounds. Exudate levels can vary markedly: Thomas *et al* (1996) and Lamke *et al* (1977) report volumes in excess of 50g per 100 cm^2 per day in both leg ulcers and burn wounds. This equates to approximately 5ml per 10 cm^2 wound area, consisting not only of fluid but also of minerals and electrolytes, particularly phosphate and magnesium (Berger *et al*, 1997).

Exudates generally have a high protein content and specific gravity (usually greater than 1.020) (Cutting and White, 2002a). Differential removal of water from exudate will concentrate solutes, particularly proteins and enzymes, and result in an increase in oncotic pressure, further favouring exudate production. Breslow (1991) has shown that patients can lose 90–100 g of protein per day in the exudate from a large cavity pressure ulcer. James *et al* (2000) indicate that low levels of protein and albumin in wound exudate, which may simply reflect patient nutritional status, can be directly linked to the likelihood of healing.

Exudate is normally pale amber in colour, but contamination by bacteria or fistula output may change this, giving a green (typically *Pseudomonas aeruginosa* infection), brown or black exudate and wound bed (*Figures 1.2* and *1.3*).

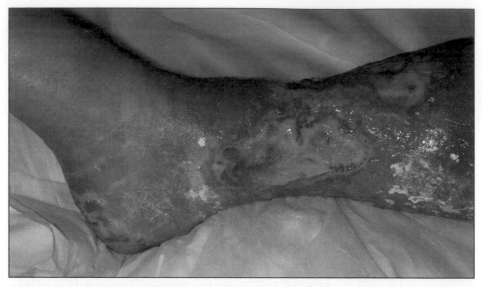

Figure 1.2: *Pseudomonas* **infection showing green wound bed and exudate**

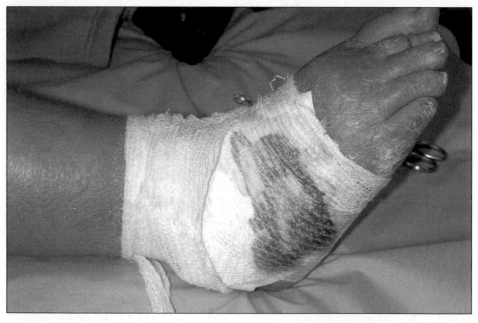

Figure 1.3: Patient at initial referral with green exudate staining dressing

Typical descriptive terms used to categorise exudate include:

⌘ Serous: clear watery consistency; exudate of this type may indicate the presence of bacteria producing a fibrinolysin, such as some strains of *Staphylococcus aureus*, ß-haemolytic group A streptococci (*Figure 1.4*)
⌘ Fibrinous: cloudy, contains fibrin protein strands.

⌘ Purulent: almost milky, containing infective bacteria and inflammatory cells.
⌘ Haemo-purulent: as above, but dermal capillary damage leads to the presence of red blood cells in the exudate.
⌘ Haemorrhagic: red blood cells are a major component of the exudate.

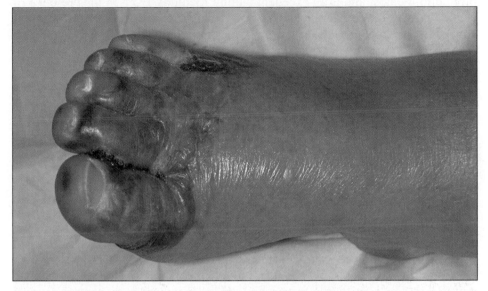

Figure 1.4: Blistering of the toes due to ß-haemolytic streptococcal infection

Acute and chronic wound exudate

In an experimental situation wound fluid from acute wounds has been demonstrated to have a beneficial effect on wound healing, stimulating fibroblast and endothelial cell production (Katz *et al*, 1991). This contrasts with the effect of chronic wound exudate, which differs markedly from exudate obtained from acute wounds (Park *et al*, 1998) in that it has an adverse effect on wound healing, slowing down or even blocking cell proliferation (Schultz *et al*, 2003).

Experimental evidence also indicates that the chronic wound environment is hypoxic, with a low glucose and high lactate content found in exudate (Nelson, 1997). Chronic wound exudate has also been shown to have a relatively high content of destructive proteinases. Palolahti *et al* (1993) have demonstrated increased proteolytic activity in the chronic ulcer exudate, a finding that differed from that in acute wound exudate from skin donor sites. A number of other authors have demonstrated similar results (Barrick *et al*, 1999; Trengove *et al*, 1999; Yager and Nwomeh, 1999).

Exudate from chronic wounds has also been shown to slow down or block the proliferation of key cells in the wound healing process (such as keratinocytes, fibroblasts and endothelial cells), to interfere with growth factor availability and to inactivate essential matrix material (Ennis and Meneses, 2000; Falanga, 2001). Drinkwater *et al* (2002) have demonstrated that venous ulcer exudate has an inhibitory effect on experimental angiogenesis. This may be related to increased proteolytic enzyme activity rather than an inadequate expression of vascular endothelial growth factor (Lauer *et al*, 2000).

The content of wound fluid does, therefore, seem to reflect the wound status and can indicate if a wound is likely to proceed to healing (Staiano-Coico *et al*, 2000). Exudate also damages the surrounding healthy skin, represents a loss of protein to the host and is an excellent culture medium. Even in the presence of clean, healthy-looking granulation tissue technologically advanced healing enhancers, such as growth factors and bioengineered skin, will perform badly if exudate is not controlled (Falanga, 2000).

It is unclear where, when or why the transition from 'favourable' acute wound fluid to 'unfavourable' chronic wound exudate occurs, but chronic wound exudate does represent a potential barrier to healing. It would appear that exudate from a non-healing chronic wound consists of a cytotoxic chemical soup capable of suppressing cell division and causing cellular death. Falanga (1992) hypothesises that the chronic wound environment is generally non-conducive to cell growth.

The composition of exudate has been discussed by Thomas (1997b). Chronic wound exudate consists of the extravascular fluid (water, salts, proteins, carbohydrate and fatty acids) plus varying quantities of cells, bacteria, cellular and bacterial debris, bacterial exotoxins and endotoxins, bacterial glycocalyx (biofilm), short-chain volatile fatty acids (which contribute to wound odour and may in themselves be cytotoxic), matrix metalloproteinases (MMPs), growth factors and free radicals. Variation in the chemical composition of an exudate will define odour, influence wound bed pH, alter wound pain, control exudate viscosity and colour, and will affect the action of the exudate on the wound bed and surrounding skin. Dressings which interact with this exudate will change the physical and chemical composition of the exudate and can, potentially, directly influence wound healing (Edwards *et al*, 1999; 2001).

Potential role of wound and exudate pH

The pH of intact skin ranges from about 4.8 to 6.0 while that of interstitial fluid exhibits a pH nearer 7.0. The low pH of the skin acts as a natural barrier to the external environment and is frequently described as 'the acid mantle' (Dikstein and Zlotogorsky, 1989).

The measurement of wound bed and therefore exudate pH has shown to be of potential value when examining the healing potential of chronic wounds. Prolonged chemical acidification of the wound bed has been shown to increase the healing rates in some wound types of chronic wounds, for example, in venous leg ulcers (Wilson *et al*, 1979). Sayegh *et al* (1988) using pH measurement was able to predict skin graft survival in an experimental and clinical study in patients with burns and chronic ulcers. The wound bed pH of both chronic venous ulcers and pressure ulcers was found to be alkaline or neutral (Mani, 1999) and has been found to change its status according to the staging of the ulcer, moving to an acidic state during healing and epithelialization (Tsukada *et al*, 1992).

Other evidence supporting the acidification of the wound bed as part of the healing process of chronic wounds includes Varghese *et al* (1986), who were able to show that acidic wound fluid collected from under synthetic dressings inhibited bacterial growth and promoted fibroblast proliferation. Moreover, Romanelli *et al* (1998) has demonstrated that the pH of a granulating wound bed changed from alkaline to acidic and was able to maintain this environment under an occlusive hydrocellular dressing.

The measurement of wound bed and exudate pH could therefore provide vital information, allowing more accurate management of the wound bed and control of the microbiological burden that is a crucial aspect in obtaining complete healing. Some wound dressings such as Promogran ™ (Johnson & Johnson) have been suggested to modify the wound bed environment by regulating proteolytic enzyme activity (Cullet *et al*, 2002) and, in so doing, also seem to influence exudate pH.

Exudate management

An understanding of the systemic and local conditions influencing exudate production and knowledge of the potentially damaging chemical constituents of exudate should inform management strategy. The management of exudate is one of the interrelated key themes developed by Falanga and others (Falanga, 2000; Sibbald, 2001; Vowden and Vowden, 2002) in the concept of 'wound bed preparation'. This concept, which has evolved to TIME, where M relates to 'moisture balance' has recently been reviewed by Schultz *et al* (2003).While this concept identifies exudate as a management pathway, it does not consider exudate management in isolation but places it in an overall wound management algorithm along with obtaining bacterial balance, the management of necrosis, the correction of cellular dysfunction and the correction of biochemical imbalance (Vowden and Vowden, 2002). Unfortunately, these fundamentals are all too often ignored, frequently with disastrous results for the patient and their immediate family (*Figures 1.5* and *1.6*).

While all wounds produce exudate, effective exudate management only forms part of the initial management strategy. Its aims can be defined as follows:

- optimizing the wound environment
- controlling infective load
- protecting the surrounding skin
- maximizing the patient's quality of life by preventing exudate leakage, controlling odour and reducing wound pain.

Exudate management strategy can be defined according to the six 'Cs' (*Box 1.1*). It starts by defining the factors that influence the production of the exudate (*Table 1.2*) and then looks at the management of the immediate clinical problem and any complications, such as skin maceration, that may have occurred. Interventions can be defined at two levels: a local (direct) level, such as the use of dressings; and a general or systemic (indirect) level, such as the use of compression bandaging to correct some of the deleterious effects of chronic venous hypertension or the use of diuretic therapy and limb elevation to manage congestive cardiac failure and peripheral oedema (*Table 1.3*).

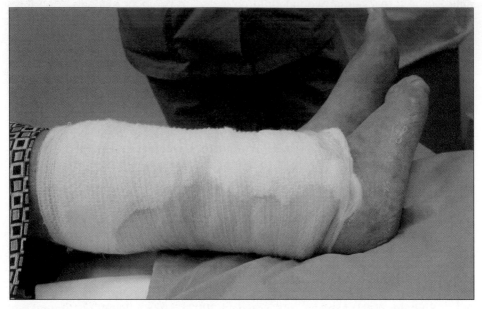

Figure 1.5: Failure of a simple but bulky dressing to control dependent drainage of exudate

Box 1.1. Exudate management strategy based on the six 'Cs'					
Cause	**Control**	**Components**	**Containment**	**Correction**	**Complications**
Systemic	Whether	Bacterial load	Dressing seal	Modification of	Skin protection
Local	effective	Necrotic tissue	Where:	bacterial load	Protein loss
Wound-	systemic or	'Chemical'	At the wound	'Debridement'	Pain
related	local control	composition	surface	Exudate	Odour
	is possible	and pH	Within the	modification	
		Viscosity and	dressing		
		volume	Away from the		
			wound		

The complications of poor exudate management may include:

- delay in healing and/or wound deterioration
- increased risk of local or systemic infection
- increased demand on nursing time and increased dressing costs
- wound surface damage
- surrounding skin damage
- failure of odour control
- detrimental effect on quality of life due to:
    ~ poor dressing fit, possibly resulting in exudate leakage
    ~ bulk of dressings
    ~ frequency of dressing change
    ~ pain.

Table 1.2: Factors that may influence exudate production (adapted from Thomas, 1997b; Cutting and White, 2002b)

Factor	Mechanism
Hydrostatic pressure	Heart failure, venous insufficiency (venous hypertension), dependency syndrome (posture)
Biochemical changes	Cellulitis, arthritis, hormonal cyclic oedema; histamine and vasoactive amines increase vascular permeability and extravasation in inflammation
Wound infection	Host inflammatory response and the action of some bacterial endo- and exotoxins which induce vascular permeability
Temperature	Increasing temperature – either systemic (pyrexia) or ambient – is associated with capillary vasodilatation
Pressure	Pressure applied either with compression bandaging or hosiery or locally to the wound bed from a dressing will decrease exudate; conversely, topical negative pressure (TNP) – though managing – may increase exudate volume
Gender	Unsubstantiated observation that males produce more exudate than women
Wound type	Type and stage of healing affect exudate levels, as does the presence of a fistula or sinus
Wound depth and surface area	Exudate levels may be up to 5 ml per 10 cm^2 wound area (see text); generally, the deeper the wound the greater the production of exudate
Type of dressing and topical treatment	Hygroscopic (Mesalt), some debriding agents and iodinated dressings may increase exudate production

Table 1.3: Levels of exudate control

Direct control	Indirect control
❖ Absorptive dressings	❖ Alleviation underlying cause

❖ Dressings modifying exudate
  • bacterial control
  • protease inhibitors
  • hyaluronic acid
	• cardiac failure
	  • dependent oedema
	  • venous disease
	  • lymphoedema

❖ Use of compression
  • static (bandages)
  • dynamic (intermittent compression therapy)	

❖ Mechanical
  • drainage
  • topical negative pressure (TNP) such as the VAC	

White (2001) has reviewed the factors involved in dressing selection when managing exudates, relating to basic dressing categories such as alginates or

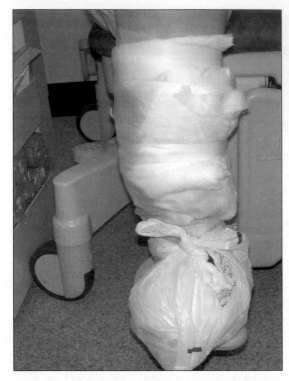

Figure 1.6: Patient modification of a bulky dressing in an attempt to control exudate

foams. We do, however, need to look beyond this and consider the effect of the dressing on the exudate and how this may affect the wound environment. The basic principles to consider are as follows:

- exudate volume
- exudate viscosity
- exudate constitution.

Dressing selection

The disproportionate absorption of any substance within the exudate will change the wound fluid constitution and therefore the wound environment. This change may be beneficial but could also be damaging as, for example, there may be depletion of co-enzymes, changes in metal ion availability (zinc), alteration in wound pH or an increase in local osmolality. All of these can potentially delay healing, although evidence supporting this hypothesis is currently lacking.

The aim of dressing use is not simply to mop up exudate, but to manage the exudate in such a way as to enhance the wound environ-ment to favour healing. *Figure 1.7* indicates the wide range of dressing functions that can be used to manage, either singly or in combination, excessive wound fluid levels. The choice of an individual product for a particular wound depends on a number of factors:

- the exudate level and the fluid-handling properties of the dressing
- whether wound fluid should be held at the wound bed or removed from it
- the site and size of the wound
- the level of contamination: bacterial or necrotic tissue
- the state of the surrounding skin
- whether the dressing is to be used in combination with other products as either a primary wound contact layer or a secondary dressing
- whether the product will be used with compression therapy.

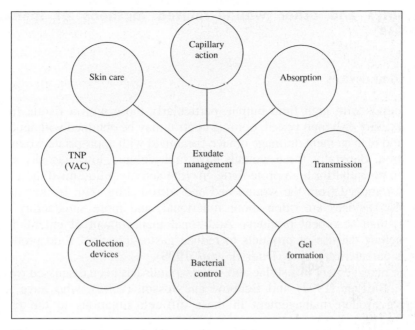

Figure 1.7: Direct methods of managing exudate

The potential exudate-handling properties of a dressing can be difficult to predict, especially as a number of different test methods have been applied. Thomas and Fram (2001) have suggested a method for dressing evaluation which facilitates direct comparisons between products that are different in structure and composition. This method may be useful in predicting the time for which dressings might be expected to remain effective on exuding wounds.

The wound care research for appropriate products (WRAP) project, a joint collaborative group with industrial and clinical partners funded by a grant from the Engineering and Physical Sciences Research Council (EPSRC) has, as part of its remit, looked specifically at dressing performance in terms of exudate handling and, in particular, exudate leakage and how it may be influenced by dressing design. This project has produced preliminary findings (Browne *et al*, 2004) and may provide improved tools for monitoring dressing performance, using TELER® (Treatment Evaluation by Le Roux's method) documentation (Le Roux, 1995; Grocott, 1998; 2000). Hopefully, these findings will inform future dressing design (Browne *et al*, 2004).

Dressings and other wound-related methods of managing exudate

Collection devices

For wounds with high fluid output, particularly those with a fistula from an enteral cavity or lymph vessel, optimal control may be obtained with an ostomy or wound management drainage device combined with appropriate wound edge protection. Generally, these wounds have high-volume, low-viscosity exudate with the potential for high proteolytic enzyme activity. Fluid must therefore be rapidly removed from the wound bed and surrounding skin. In this situation collection devices are often more functional, and more satisfactory to the patient, than absorbent products. Additional management of enteral fistulae may include the use of products to reduce gastro-intestinal fluid production, such as parenteral feeding (Dudrick *et al*, 1999).

The management of fistulae and sinus wounds has been discussed by Black (1995), Butcher (1999) and Benbow and Iosson (2002), who have related effective exudate management in these difficult situations to the patient's quality of life.

Capillary action dressings

These dressings conduct fluid away from the wound surface. They are usually multi-layered, with the inner, non-adherent layer conducting the fluid vertically. Subsequent layers hold and dissipate the fluid throughout the outer component of the compound dressing (*Figure 1.8*).

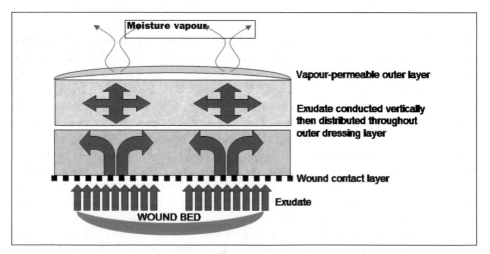

Figure 1.8: Capillary action dressings

These dressings have been shown to be effective in wounds with moderate to high exudate volumes of low to moderate viscosity (Russell *et al*, 2001; Deeth, 2002).

Cadexomer beads can function in a similar way, with fluid being taken into the beads along an osmotic gradient and away from the wound surface (Marzin, 1993). Iodine is released from some cadexomer products (Hansson, 1998).

Absorptive dressings

These dressings consist of foam or a pad with a primary non-adherent wound contact layer. They can handle moderate to high volumes of fluid but do not manage high-viscosity exudate well.

The foam dressings fall into two basic categories: a simple foam and a foam dressing incorporating a vapour-permeable film backing, which allows evaporation of fluid from the dressing surface (*Figure 1.9*).

These dressings have

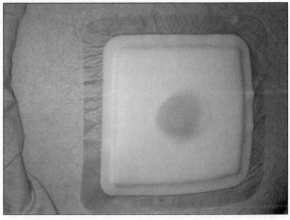

Figure 1.9: Foam dressing used to manage a moderately exudating pressure ulcer

been shown to be effective in a number of wound types (Collier, 1992; Thomas, 1997b, c; Taylor *et al*, 1999). However, dressing absorptive capacity can be compromised under pressure, such as when used with high-compression bandaging.

Transmission dressings

These dressings manage fluid load by allowing evaporation of volatile components, such as water vapour from the dressing surface; the remainder of the exudate is held next to the wound. This fluid loss is recorded as the dressing moisture vapour transmission rate (MVTR).

Most laboratory work in this field has been in the assessment of film dressings (Thomas, 1996; Thomas *et al*, 1997). The selective release of water vapour can result in a concentration of the other, potentially damaging, components within the exudates, some of which may be held at the wound surface. These dressings are therefore most suitable for acute wounds with low to moderate exudate volumes of low viscosity, although they have been shown to be of value in high-volume, low-viscosity exuding malignant wounds (Grocott, personal communication).

Some dressings combine the action of transmission and absorbency into a single composite dressing. This increases the volume of exudate such dressings can handle and holds the 'concentrated' exudate within the absorbent layer.

Gel formation dressing

One component of the dressing — frequently a hydrocolloid, hydrogel, alginate or hydrofibre — takes up fluid to form a gel. This gel is then held within the dressing but in contact with the wound surface, facilitating autolytic debridement.

Depending on the formulation, hydrocolloids and hydrogels can either absorb exudate or rehydrate a wound and are most suitable for wounds with a low to moderate volume of exudate of moderate to high viscosity (*Figure 1.10*). Alginate (Stewart, 2002) and hydrofibre dressings are suitable for moderate to high volumes of exudate with moderate to high viscosity (*Figure 1.11*).

Hydrofibres have been shown to be effective in heavily exudating acute (Foster and Moore, 1997; Robinson, 2000) and chronic wounds (Armstrong and Ruckley, 1997). Their relatively pain-free removal can be an advantage (Moore and Foster, 2000). Depending on the formulation of the product, other elements within the exudate (such as bacteria or MMPs) may be absorbed or modified (Stewart, 2002).

Bacterial control dressing

Products containing iodine (European Tissue Repair Society [ETRS], 1995; Gilchrist, 1997) and silver can, through their antiseptic or antimicrobial action, reduce the bacterial load (Stewart, 2002) and subsequent exudate levels. Such dressings are suitable for moderately to heavily exudating (high-volume and viscosity) wounds with evidence of heavy bacterial colonization or overt infection.

The (in vitro) antimicrobial effects of silver-containing dressings have been reviewed by Thomas and McCubbin (2003). The wider role of silver has been reviewed by several authors (Demling and DeSanti, 2001; Lansdown, 2002a, b), as has the role of iodine and its impact on wound physiology (ETRS, 1995).

These dressings often have an additional debriding action and function well when used in combination with compression therapy in the management of the ulcerated oedematous limb.

Topical negative pressure

The use of topical negative pressure (TNP) with devices such as the VAC (Vacuum-Assisted Closure, KCI) has been shown to be effective in the management of a variety of acute and chronic wounds (Deva *et al*, 1997; Mullner *et al*, 1997; Mendez-Eastman, 1998).

This form of therapy is suitable for high-volume, low- to high-viscosity exudate. It has been suggested that this device reduces bacterial load (Morykwas et al, 1997), but benefits may also accrue from the removal of bacterial toxins, MMPs and other toxic chemicals from the wound environment.

The negative pressure may also encourage angiogenesis and the development of healthy granulation tissue (Voinchet and Magalon, 1996). It should be noted, however, that a case report (Chester and Waters, 2002) indicates that there could be a potential for anaerobic infection to develop under TNP. This suggests that wounds need to be carefully monitored while undergoing this form of therapy for exudate management.

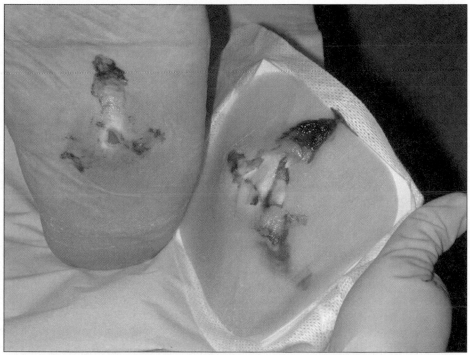

Figure 1.10: Hydrocolloid dressing used to manage a low-exudating ulcer on the sole of a foot

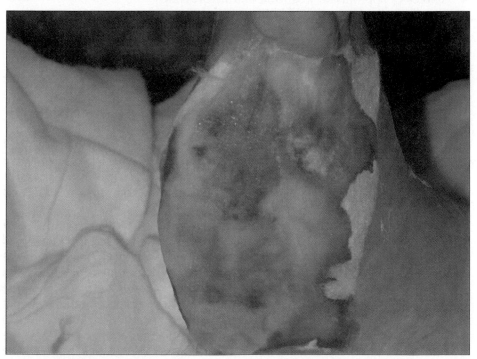

Figure 1.11: Alginate used to manage moderate- to high-volume and high-viscosity exudate immediately prior to removal

Surrounding skin care

The skin around a chronic wound is at risk of maceration and contact dermatitis, particularly in the presence of high exudate output (Cutting, 1999; Nielsen, 1999; Cutting and White, 2002a, b). Periwound skin has also been shown to be more highly susceptible to damage as its barrier integrity is compromised (Walker *et al*, 1997).

Care of the surrounding skin is therefore an integral part of exudate management. This is particularly important where healing is unlikely to occur because of other elements, such as bile or digestive juices contaminate the exudate or where the surrounding skin is already damaged or friable, such as after radiotherapy or steroid treatment. The skin protection policy should include the following:

- skin care at dressing change
- selection of the appropriate dressing type to manage the volume and type of exudate
- careful application of one or more dressings of the appropriate size
- the establishment of a good dressing seal, taking into consideration other requirements such as movement
- understanding of the adhesive properties of the dressing and how to remove it
- recognition that the adhesive component of the dressing may further damage and macerate the periwound skin
- choice of appropriate wear time for the dressing
- protection of the surrounding skin by the use of barrier cream, spray film or masking. The use of these products is under-researched, but their use has been discussed by several authors (Dealey, 1999; Briggs and Torra i Bou, 2002; Cutting and White, 2002b).

Conclusion

Effective management of wound exudate is one of the cornerstones of good wound care. Changes in the volume and nature of exudate provide valuable information on the underlying state of the wound (Nelson, 1997) and may give an indication of an increasing bacterial load and the presence of infection (Cutting and White, 2002b).

As fundamental differences exist between acute and chronic wound exudates, management strategies will need to vary according to the wound type. Chronic wound exudate should be regarded as a 'wounding' agent with the ability to destroy tissue (Chen, 1998). So, while the principle of moist wound healing must be adhered to, a balance must be achieved and the potential harmful effects of chronic wound exudate neutralized, either by modifying the exudate or by removing the exudate from the wound surface.

Changes in wound exudate reflect the state of the underlying wound and the general health of the patient. Careful monitoring of the exudate can provide valuable information for the application of systemic and local therapies. Individual wound care products have specific functions which relate to the volume, viscosity and nature of the exudate. These functions should provide a guide to the selection of skin care and dressings for the management of different wound types.

> **Key points**
>
> ⌘ Fundamental differences exist between acute and chronic wound exudates.
>
> ⌘ Management strategies need to vary according to the wound type.
>
> ⌘ Dressing selection needs to match product properties with wound characteristics.

References

Armstrong SH, Ruckley CV (1997) Use of a fibrous dressing in exuding leg ulcers. *J Wound Care* **6**(7): 322–4

Baker EA, Leaper DJ (2000) Proteinases, their inhibitors, and cytokine profiles in acute wound fluid. *Wound Repair Regen* **8**(5): 392–8

Barrick B, Campbell EJ, Owen CA (1999) Leukocyte proteinases in wound healing: roles in physiologic and pathologic processes. *Wound Repair Regen* **7**(6): 410–22

Benbow M, Iosson G (2002) Fistula management following an appendicectomy: nursing challenges. *J Wound Care* **11**(2): 59–61

Berger MM, Rothen C, Cavadini C, Chiolero RL (1997) Exudative mineral losses after serious burns: a clue to the alterations of magnesium and phosphate metabolism. *Am J Clin Nutr* **65**(5): 1473–81

Bishop SM, Walker M, Rogers AA, Chen WY (2003) Importance of moisture balance at the wound-dressing interface. *J Wound Care* **12**(4): 125–8

Black PK (1995) Caring for large wounds and fistulas. *J Wound Care* **4**(1): 23–6

Bolton LL, Monte K, Pirone LA (2000) Moisture and healing: beyond the jargon. *Ostomy Wound Manage* **46**(1A Suppl): S51–62; quiz S63–4

Breslow R (1991) Nutritional status and dietary intake of patients with pressure ulcers: review of research literature 1943 to 1989. *Decubitus* **4**(1): 16–21

Briggs M, Torra i Bou JE (2002) Pain at wound dressing changes: a guide to management. In: Moffatt, C ed. *Pain at wound dressing change*. Medical Education Partnership, London: 12–17

Browne N, Grocott P, Cowley S, Cameron J, Dealey C, Keogh A *et al* (2004) Woundcare Research for Appropriate Products (WRAP): validation of the TELER method involving users. *Int J Nurs Stud* **41**(5): 559–71

Buchan IA, Andrews JK, Lang SM (1980) Clinical and laboratory investigation of the composition and properties of human skin wound exudate under semi-permeable dressings. *Burns* **7**: 326–34

Butcher M (1999) Management of wound sinuses. *J Wound Care* **8**(9): 451–4

Chen J (1998) *Aquacel hydrofibre dressing: The next step in wound dressing technology*. ConvaTec, London

Chester DL, Waters R (2002) Adverse alteration of wound flora with topical negative-pressure therapy: a case report. *Br J Plast Surg* **55**(6): 510–11

Collier J (1992) A moist, odour-free environment. A multicentred trial of a foamed gel and a hydrocolloid dressing. *Prof Nurse* **7**(12): 804–8

Cullen B, Smith R, McCulloch E, Silcock D, Morrison L (2002) Mechanism of action of PROMOGRAN, a protease modulating matrix, for the treatment of diabetic foot ulcers. *Wound Repair Regen* **10**: 16–25

Cutting KF (1999) The causes and prevention of maceration of the skin. *J Wound Care* **8**(4): 200–1

Cutting KF, White RJ (2002a) Maceration of the skin and wound bed. 1: Its nature and causes. *J Wound Care* **11**(7): 275–8

Cutting KF, White RJ (2002b) Avoidance and management of peri-wound maceration of the skin. *Prof Nurse* **18**(1): 33–6

Dealy C (1999) *The Care of Wounds: A Guide for Nurses.* 2nd edn. Blackwell Science, London

Deeth M (2002) Review of an independent audit into the clinical efficacy of VACUTEX. *Br J Nurs* **11**(12 Suppl): S60, S62–6

Demling RH, DeSanti L (2001) The role of silver technology in wound healing Part 1: Effect of silver on wound management. *Wounds: A compendium of clinical Research and Practice* **13**(1 (Supplement A): 4–15

Deva AK, Siu C, Nettle WJ (1997) Vacuum-assisted closure of a sacral pressure sore. *J Wound Care* **6**(7): 311–12

Dikstein S, Zlotogorsky A (1989) In: Leveque JL, ed. Cutaneous *Investigations in Health and Disease — Non-invasive Methods and Instruments.* Marcel Dekker, New York: 59–62

Drinkwater SL, Smith A, Sawyer BM, Burnand KG (2002) Effect of venous ulcer exudates on angiogenesis in vitro. *Br J Surg* **89**(6): 709–13

Dudrick SJ, Maharaj AR, McKelvey AA (1999) Artificial nutritional support in patients with gastrointestinal fistulas. *World J Surg* **23**(6): 570–6

Edwards JV, Bopp AF, Batiste S *et al* (1999) Inhibition of elastase by a synthetic cotton-bound serine protease inhibitor: in vitro kinetics and inhibitor release. *Wound Repair Regen* **7**(2): 106–18

Edwards JV, Yager DR, Cohen IK *et al* (2001) Modified cotton gauze dressings that selectively absorb neutrophil elastase activity in solution. *Wound Repair Regen* **9**(1): 50–8

Ennis WJ, Meneses P (2000) Wound healing at the local level: The stunned wound. *Ostomy Wound Manage* **46**(1A Suppl): 39S–48S

European Tissue Repair Society (1995) Iodine and wound physiology: a symposium. In: Hunt T, Middlekoop E, eds. *Proceedings of 5th Annual Meeting of the European Tissue Repair Society.* ETRS, Padua

Falanga V (1992) Growth factors and chronic wounds: the need to understand the microenvironment. *J Dermatol* **19**(11): 667–72

Falanga V (2000) Classifications for wound bed preparation and stimulation of chronic wounds. *Wound Repair Regen* **8**(5): 347–52

Falanga V (2001) Introducing the concept of wound bed preparation. *An International Forum on Wound Care* **16**(1): 1–4

Foster L, Moore P (1997) The application of a cellulose-based fibre dressing in surgical wounds. *J Wound Care* **6**(10): 469–73

Gilchrist B (1997) Should iodine be reconsidered in wound management? European Tissue Repair Society. *J Wound Care* **6**(3): 148–50Grocott P (1997) Evaluation of a tool used to assess the management of fungating wounds. *J Wound Care* **6**(9): 421–4

Grocott P (1998) Exudate management in fungating wounds. *J Wound Care* **7**(9): 445–8

Grocott P (2000) The palliative management of fungating malignant wounds. *J Wound Care* **9**(1): 4–9

Hansson, C (1997) Interactive wound dressings. A practical guide to their use in older patients. *Drugs Aging* **11**(4): 271–84

Hansson C (1998) The effects of cadexomer iodine paste in the treatment of venous leg ulcers compared with hydrocolloid dressing and paraffin gauze dressing. Cadexomer Iodine Study Group. *Int J Dermatol* **37**(5): 390–6

James TJ, Hughes MA, Cherry GW, Taylor RP (2000) Simple biochemical markers to assess chronic wounds. *Wound Repair Regen* **8**(4): 264–9

Katz MH, Alvarez AF, Kirsner RS, Eaglstein WH, Falanga V (1991) Human wound fluid from acute wounds stimulates fibroblast and endothelial cell growth. *J Am Acad Dermatol* **25**(6 Pt 1): 1054–8

Lamke LO, Nilsson GE, Reichner HL (1977) The evaporative water loss from burns and water vapour permeability of grafts and artificial membranes used in the treatment of burns. *Burns* **3**: 159–65

Lansdown AB (2002a) Silver 1: Its antibacterial properties and mechanism of action. *J Wound Care* **11**(4): 125–30

Lansdown AB (2002b) Silver 2: Toxicity in mammals and how its products aid wound repair. *J Wound Care* **11**(5): 173–7

Lauer G, Sollberg S, Cole M *et al* (2000) Expression and proteolysis of vascular endothelial growth factor is increased in chronic wounds. *J Invest Dermatol* **115**(1): 12–8

Le Roux A (1995) TELER: The concept. *Physiotherapy* **79**(11): 755–8

Mani R (1999) Science of measurements in wound healing. *J Wound Repair Regen* **7**(5): 330–4

Marzin L (1993) Comparing dextranomer absorbent pads and dextranomer paste in the treatment of venous leg ulcers. *J Wound Care* **2**(2): 80–3

Mendez-Eastman S (1998) Negative pressure wound therapy. *Plast Surg Nurs* **18**(1): 27–9, 33–7

Moore K (1999) Cell biology of chronic wounds: the role of inflammation. *J Wound Care* **8**(7): 345–8

Moore PJ, Foster L (2000) Cost benefits of two dressings in the management of surgical wounds. *Br J Nurs* **9**(17): 1128–32

Morykwas MJ, Argenta LC, Shelton-Brown EI, McGuirt W (1997) Vacuum-assisted closure: a new method for wound control and treatment: animal studies and basic foundation. *Ann Plast Surg* **38**(6): 553–62

Mullner T, Mrkonjic L, Kwasny O, Vecsei V (1997) The use of negative pressure to promote the healing of tissue defects: a clinical trial using the vacuum sealing technique. *Br J Plast Surg* **50**(3): 194–9

Nelson EA (1997) Is exudate a clinical problem: a nurse's perspective? In: Cherry G, Harding K, eds. *Management of Wound Exudates*. SOFOS, Oxford: 11–12

Nielsen A (1999) Management of wound exudate. *Br J Community Nurs* **13**(6): 27–34

Ovens N, Fairhurst J (2002) Management of a heavily exuding, painful wound with necrotising subcutaneous infection. *J Wound Care* **11**(1): 25–7

Palolahti M, Lauharanta J, Stephens RW, Kuusela P, Vaheri A (1993) Proteolytic activity in leg ulcer exudate. *Exp Dermatol* **2**(1): 29–37

Park HY, Shon K, Phillips T (1998) The effect of heat on the inhibitory effects of chronic wound fluid on fibroblasts *in vitro*. *Wounds* **10**: 189–92

Partsch H (2003) Understanding the pathophysiological effects of compression. In: Moffatt C, ed. *Position Paper: Understanding Compression Therapy*. MEP, London

Robinson BJ (2000) The use of a hydrofibre dressing in wound management. *J Wound Care* **9**(1): 32–4

Romanelli M, Schipani E, Paiaggesi A, Barachini P (1998) In: Suggett A, Cherry G, Mani R, Agstein W, eds. *International Congress Symposium Series*. Royal Society of medicine Press, London: 57–61

Russell L, Deeth M, Jones HM, Reynolds T (2001) VACUTEX capillary action dressing: a multicentre, randomized trial. *Br J Nurs* **10**(11 Suppl): S66–70

Sayegh N, Dawson J, Bloom N, Stahl W (1988) Wound pH as a predictor of skin graft survival. *Curr Surg* **45**: 23–4

Schultz GS, Sibbald RG, Falanga V *et al* (2003) Wound bed preparation: a systematic approach to wound management. *Wound Repair Regen* **11**(Suppl 1): S1–S28

Sibbald, RG (2001) What is the bacterial burden of the wound bed and does it matter? In: Cherry GW, Harding KG, Ryan TJ, eds. *Wound Bed Preparation*. Royal Society of Medicine Press, London: 41–50

Staiano-Coico L, Higgins PJ, Schwartz SB, Zimm AJ, Goncalves J (2000) Wound fluids: a reflection of the state of healing. *Ostomy Wound Manage* **46**(1A Suppl): S85–93; quiz S94–5

Stewart J (2002) *Next generation products for wound management*. World Wide Wounds. Online at: http://www.worldwidewounds.com (accessed August 2003)

Taylor A, Lane C, Walsh J, Whittaker S, Ballard K, Young SR (1999) A non-comparative multi-centre clinical evaluation of a new hydropolymer adhesive dressing. *J Wound Care* **8**(10): 489–92

Thomas S (1996) Vapour-permeable film dressings. *J Wound Care* **5**(6): 271–4

Thomas S (1997a) Exudate: who needs it? In: Cherry G, Harding K, eds. *Management of Wound Exudate*. SOFOS, Oxford: 1–4

Thomas S (1997b) Assessment and management of wound exudate. *J Wound Care* **6**(7): 327–30

Thomas S (1997c) A guide to dressing selection. *J Wound Care* **6**(10): 479–82

Thomas S, Banks V, Fear M, Hagelstein S, Bale S, Harding K (1997) A study to compare two film dressings used as secondary dressings. *J Wound Care* **6**(7): 333–6

Thomas S, Fear M, Humphreys J, Disley L, Waring MJ (1996) The effect of dressings on the production of exudate from venous leg ulcers. *Wounds* **8**(5): 145–50

Thomas S, Fram P (2001) The development of a novel technique for predicting the exudate handling properties of modern wound dressings. *J Tissue Viabil* **11**(4): 145–53, 156–60

Thomas S, McCubbin P (2003) A comparison of the antimicrobial effects of four silver-containing dressings on three organisms. *J Wound Care* **12**(3): 101–7

Tsukada K, Tokunaga K, Iwama T, Mishima Y (1992) The pH changes of pressure ulcers relates to the healing process of wounds. *Wounds* **4**: 16–20

Trengove NJ, Stacey MC, MacAuley S *et al* (1999) Analysis of the acute and chronic wound environments: the role of proteases and their inhibitors. *Wound Repair Regen* **7**(6): 442–52

Varghese MC, Balin AK, Carter DM, Caldwell D (1986) Local environment of chronic wounds under synthetic dressings. *Arch Dermatol* **122**: 52–7

Vogt PM, Andree C, Breuing K et al (1995) Dry, moist, and wet skin wound repair. *Ann Plast Surg* **34**(5): 493–9, discussion 499–500

Voinchet V, Magalon G (1996) Vacuum assisted closure. Wound healing by negative pressure. *Ann Chir Plast Esthet* **41**(5): 583–9

Vowden P, Vowden K (2002) *Wound bed preparation*. World Wide Wounds. Online at: http://www.worldwidewounds.com/2002/april/Vowden/Wound-Bed-Preparation.html

Walker M, Hulme TA, Rippon MG *et al* (1997) In vitro model(s) for the percutaneous delivery of active tissue repair agents. *J Pharm Sci* **86**(12): 1379–84

Watret L (1997) Know how... management of wound exudate. *Nurs Times* **93**(30): 38–9

White R (2001) Managing exudate. *Nurs Times* **97**(9): XI–XIII

Wilson IA, Henry M, Quill RD, Byrne PJ (1979) The pH of varicose ulcer surfaces and its relationship to healing. *Vasa* **8**: 339–42

Winter GD (1962) Formation of the scab and the rate of epithelization of superficial wounds in the skin of the young domestic pig. *Nature* **193**(4812): 293–4

Yager DR, Nwomeh BC (1999) The proteolytic environment of chronic wounds. *Wound Repair Regen* **7**(6): 433–41

2

Maceration of the skin and wound bed by indication

Richard J White, Keith F Cutting

In the course of managing wounds, particularly exuding chronic wounds, failure to manage adequately exudate can lead to exposure of the peri-wound skin to exudate and hence damage. This results in maceration of the skin and wound bed. Maceration is a largely under-recognized problem and one of the causes of delayed wound healing. This chapter describes a wide variety of wounds and skin conditions in which maceration might be present, or develop, during treatment, together with some strategies for avoiding maceration and the evidence base supporting them. It is only by becoming familiar with the various presentations of maceration, and with prophylactic treatment measures, that practitioners can avoid the associated morbidity and increased costs.

Maceration is a wound care management problem that has received only scant attention in the literature, apart from contributions by Cutting (1999) and Cutting and White (2002b) and White and Cutting (2003). These articles presented an overview or summary of the problem, while Cutting and White (2002a) provided an in-depth review of the literature, encompassing aetiology and the management of maceration. This chapter provides an additional perspective, detailing maceration in a variety of wound types and suggesting interventions to prevent its occurrence.

Dressings (medical devices) are the first line of approach when managing chronic wounds. Clinicians have witnessed an evolutionary change over the past twenty years, not only in the choice of dressings available but also, and more importantly, in the way that dressings interact with the wound environment.

The choice of dressings available ranges from the simple low adherent interface with the wound to what some commentators have described as 'intelligent dressings' (Palamand *et al*, 1992; Bishop *et al*, 2003). Intelligent dressings are those that have the capability to alter their moisture vapour transmission rate (MVTR) in accordance with exudate levels, thus maintaining a constant moist wound environment. Although the choice of dressing should be based on the needs of the wound bed, this should not be the sole consideration when selecting a dressing. Attention should also be paid to achieving the correct, or 'optimum', moisture balance at the interface of wound and dressing (Bishop *et al*, 2003).

Dressings also have a prophylactic and therapeutic role to play in the care of the peri-wound skin (Thomas, 1997), which may become damaged by fluid exuding from the wound (Cutting and White, 2002b). It is also possible that some dressings may help to reduce friction and provide skin protection in patients at risk of pressure area damage (Bennett and Moody, 1995a). In addition, care of the peri-wound skin can be supported not only by 'orthodox' dressings but also by products such as moisturizers (Aqueous Cream BP) and skin barriers, eg. SuperSkin™ (Clini-Med) or Cavilon™ (3M Health Care) (Hampton and Collins, 2001). Additionally, ancillary products may augment protection of the peri-wound skin, or dry up wet wounds, eg. eosin and dilute potassium permanganate solutions, although there is little or no evidence to support this notion.

The risk of skin breakdown increases with age, physical frailty, reduced mobility and incontinence (Springett and White, 2003). Maceration may be a factor in this type of skin breakdown and a feature of delayed healing in acute wound healing, but it is more likely to be a component of a chronic wound (Cutting and White, 2002a). *Figure 2.1* shows maceration evident around a venous leg ulcer.

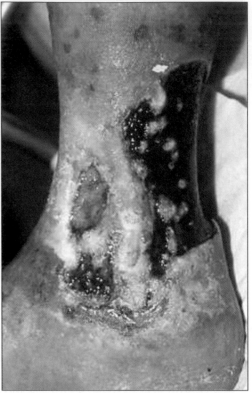

Figure 2.1: Maceration evident around a venous leg ulcer

Maceration is a function of exudate in most instances; therefore, one has to look at factors that influence the generation of exudate and indirect factors, the effects of which can control exudate generation. These factors will influence the development of maceration; examples include compression (for venous leg ulcers) and topical antimicrobials and systemic antibiotics that reduce the bacterial bioburden (White, 2001), and hence exudate production.

The choice of intervention should reflect level and consistency of exudate, and site and condition of the wound (White, 2001; Jones, 2004). It is important not to exceed the wear time beyond that within which the dressing is able to cope adequately with the production of exudate. It is also important to remember that exudate (and hence maceration) of venous leg ulcers can be controlled with compression therapy and elevation of the limb where clinically indicated (Cutting, 1999). Additionally, zinc paste bandages, zinc oxide paste BP, and '50/50' (a mixture of 50% white soft paraffin and 50% liquid paraffin) all provide valuable protection for the skin by acting as barrier agents (Cameron, 1998). Patch testing before application is advisable to avoid unwanted sensitivity reactions (Newton and Cameron, 2003).

A deteriorating (ie. enlarging) wound indicates the need for evaluation of management, and careful assessment of the wound and estimation of exudate levels at every dressing change (Flanagan, 1996). If the wound is static or deteriorating, it is important to consider the presence of infection. Switching the dressing for no objective reason should be avoided. Highly absorbent dressings, such as alginates, may be used to cover the peri-ulcer area generously, and absorbent pads may be employed as secondary dressing to provide additional absorption (Thomas, 1998).

The use of corticosteroids (for their anti-inflammatory and vasoconstrictive actions) in this situation generates heated debate. They appear to be of benefit in the management of leg ulcers, chiefly on the peri-ulcer skin when wet eczema is present (Cameron, 1998), but there does not appear to be any evidence to support their use on the wound bed.

Risks and treatment of maceration by indication

It is accepted that there are significant differences in the skin, related to age, gender and body location. The condition of the skin also varies, eg. skin may be naturally dry or greasy/oily, damp, thin and tissue-like or normal. It is likely that all of these features will be relevant to the development of maceration and/or skin breakdown. The amount of objective evidence available on maceration is very limited; there have been few studies evaluating the clinical efficacy of prophylactic treatments, such as skin protectants (Cameron *et al*, 2003; Cameron and Newton, 2003), or treatments for existing maceration.

Good clinical practice should aim to avoid maceration by prophylaxis, rather than treat it when it occurs. The maintenance of good skin condition around lesions such as wounds, fistulas and stomas is a constant concern for clinical carers. The frequent use of tapes and adhesive dressings, and exposure to exudate and effluent, represent a serious insult to skin integrity (Rottmann *et al*, 1993; Dykes and Heggie, 2001; 2003). Products available for skin protection (prophylaxis) include films, barrier ointments, emulsifiers and liquid polymers.

Before considering the application of any dressing it is important to address the root cause of the lesion, eg. apply graduated external compression in a patient with venous insufficiency, and aim to relieve or avoid pressure in an individual with pressure ulcers. All infections should be treated appropriately, including fungal infections, and sinuses and/or fistulas should be corrected surgically. Incontinence must also be taken into account, and secure and effective appliances for urostomy and/or ileostomy must be provided.

The next step is to treat any underlying medical problems, taking care to control the wound bioburden before addressing the immediate wound issues such as debridement and selection of appropriate dressing (Vowden and Vowden, 2003).

General rules of wound management to avoid or reduce maceration

The following rules are suggested to avoid or reduce maceration:

⌘ Select dressing(s) according to the level of exudate — as a rule, select highly absorbent dressings, such as alginates, hydropolymer ('plus' variant), hydrofibre and hydrofibre/hydrocolloid for heavily exuding wounds (some of these dressings can be used in multiple layers if required); use absorbent pads and tape to secure. There is anecdotal evidence that iodinated dressings 'dry up' wet wounds. This could be due to their antibacterial effect — some wound bacteria are known to provoke exudate, even in pre-infected states. For moderately exuding wounds, use dressings such as 'regular' hydropolymer and polyurethane foams, and hydrocolloid. Where skin trauma is evident or possible, take care with adhesive dressings. For lightly exuding wounds, use 'Lite' hydropolymer and foam, or thin hydrocolloid. Highly absorbent dressings can be used effectively on moderate or lightly exuding wounds to provide longer wear times. The secondary (retaining) dressing will also have an impact on wear time (Thomas, 1998).

⌘ Estimate the optimal wear time as objectively as possible. By definition, heavily exuding wounds will mean short wear times (no more than twenty-four hours); prolonging this will increase the likelihood of maceration. Moderately exuding wounds dressed with absorbent dressings may be left for up to five days between dressing changes. These are suggested guidelines and should not be taken as substantiation for evidence-based practice. Clinical judgment should be the only basis for anticipating wear time. It is preferable to err on the side of caution and not to prolong wear time for expediency. Expect wear time to increase as the wound heals, and to decrease when infection arises.

⌘ Recognize and treat any infections; expect to see increased exudate and anticipate reduced wear time in the presence of infection, even with absorbent dressings.

⌘ Use compression therapy and recommend elevation for appropriate leg ulcers.

Burns

Burns can generate very high levels of exudate (Lamke *et al*, 1997), and these may have deleterious effects on local tissues. High local water levels, achieved through excess wound exudate, will tend to encourage the growth of water-loving bacteria such as *Pseudomonas spp*. The growth of *Pseudomonas aeruginosa* has been shown to require a high water activity (which is a way of expressing the amount of free water available for bacterial growth, thus an a_w of 1 is 100% available free water) (a_w 0.97) for growth; in practice this equates to a 'wet wound' with serous exudate (Orth, 1993). Thus, the early management of burns should include measures to reduce exudate levels. Absorbent dressings, such as alginates, have proven useful for the management of exuding minor burns (Thomas, 1992).

Diabetic foot ulcers

People with diabetes may develop chronic non-healing wounds on their feet (Springett and White, 2003) as a result of the pathology underlying the diabetes. These wounds may become macerated from copious exudate and require regular changes of absorbent dressings. Additionally, the plantar surface of the foot may become very moist, and care is required to keep the skin between the toes dry to avoid fungal infections. *Figure 2.2* shows maceration of the plantar skin.

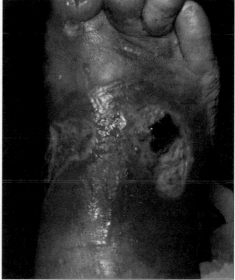

Figure 2.2: Plantar surface maceration visible on the right border (dorsal view)

Donor sites

Donor site wounds heal by secondary intent, ie. re-epithelialization of the harvested area. Donor sites are well known for their copious exudate production (Fowler and Dempsey, 1998). Although thin split-thickness sites will heal without complication in most patients, there are management problems associated with the exudate. A dry site with too little exudate and a wet site with too much can both compromise healing. The 'ideal' donor site dressing has been defined by Fowler and Dempsey (1998) and a modified set of criteria is shown in *Table 2.1*.

Many dressings have been evaluated on donor sites as this is a useful acute wound model. Films (James and Watson, 1975), paraffin gauzes (Alexander *et al*, 1983; Feldman, 1991), hydrocolloids (Brotherston and Lawrence, 1993), alginates (Brady *et al*, 1980; Attwood, 1989) and hydrofibre (Jakobsson and Bjorklund, 2000) have all been found to be of some value, with certain dressings, notably alginates, proving superior to traditional dressings (Brady *et al*, 1980). However, it would appear that gauzes remain the mainstay of donor site treatment despite their shortcomings.

Table 2.1: Criteria for the ideal donor site dressing
Reduces pain
Easy to apply and remove
Controls exudate
Promotes rapid healing
Avoids morbidity
Cost-effective
Permits easy access/observation of wound

modified from Fowler and Dempsey, 1998

Eczema

Eczema is a generic term, synonymous with 'dermatitis', for a group of inflammatory skin conditions characterized by pruritus. The group is large and includes acute and chronic conditions of intrinsic/endogenous or extrinsic/exogenous origin. The reader is referred to a review by Leung and Bieber (2003) for details of nomenclature and pathophysiology. Most eczematous conditions, and notably atopic dermatitis, are associated with abnormal skin lipid metabolism. This leads to an impaired skin barrier function which results in the leakage of serous fluid on to the skin surface (White *et al*, 1990; Imokawa, 2001). Although control of this exudate is not the primary objective of treatment, some form of absorptive dressing is necessary in order to 'neutralize' the effects of serum proteases that might provoke itching and excoriation (Newton and Cameron, 2003).

Fistulas

A fistula is a tract that develops between a vessel, body cavity or the skin. Fistulas can appear at any site of the body, present complex management problems and are likely to require multiprofessional solutions (Metcalf, 1999). In terms of wound management, those that open on to the skin (enterocutaneous fistulas) are the ones that present challenges to the tissue viability practitioner.

One definition of a wound is 'a physical injury to the body consisting of a laceration or breaking of the skin or mucous membrane' (MEDLINEplus, 2002). This definition may at first seem inappropriate when considering a fistula, but the tissue through which the fistula has formed has suffered an assault from the products of inflammation or infection. An abscess may or may not be implicated in this process. Fistulas are usually infected tracts, and some effluent will be produced. In this instance, the effluent (liquid waste leaving its source) is the wound fluid and will drain from the distal body cavity. Hence, the major component(s) of this wound fluid will be neither exudative nor transudative in origin.

For the purpose of management, fistulas may be regarded as chronic wounds. Enterocutaneous fistulae are abnormal joins between the skin and GI tract (Burch, 2004). The main aims are to keep the lesion comfortable for the patient, and odourless, to promote healing and avoid deterioration, and to help generate a positive body image. Fluid originating from an internal organ, especially the small bowel, will have a low pH and contain digestive enzymes. If these enzymes come into contact with the skin, excoriation and erosion will result. If the integrity of the skin is breached the risk of maceration arises. Although this may be of lower significance, aiming to prevent it will help to avoid more noteworthy adverse events.

Stoma appliances are suitable for collecting effluent from bowel–skin fistulas (Burch, 2004). The application of barrier sealants will provide additional protection for the skin and help to maintain its integrity, while also guaranteeing an efficient seal between the flange of the appliance and the skin. Generating a tailor-made dressing produces a result that fits the wound exactly. An inexpensive dressing pad may be all that is required to assist in retaining the dressing in the fistula (Collier, 2003; Fletcher, 2003). The important topic of skin problems around fistulae and stomata, arising from trauma, disease and maceration has been reviewed by Burch (2004).

Fungal infections

As it does with the growth of many microorganisms, a high local water content will tend to encourage the growth of fungi (Burns, 1998), particularly fungi in the dermatophyte group and yeasts. Candida albicans infection occurs in infants as napkin candidiasis and in elderly people as intertrigo (McMahon, 1994). In each case, the tissues are moist and the infection leads to redness, pain and further damage (McMahon, 1994).

Appropriate antifungal agents are the optimum treatment. Dusting powders, such as talc, are not effective as they tend to 'cake' and act as foci for further trauma (McMahon, 1994).

Fungating wounds

The management of fungating wounds is a complex task and the practitioner is faced with a number of challenges. Such wounds may present with malodour, high levels of exudate, pain, and a disturbing visual appearance, together with the certainty that they will not heal (Naylor, 2002). Enhancing quality of life through symptom control is a major issue in care, but the edict of addressing the root cause (above) is not necessarily achievable in this instance.

Fungating tumours may produce a considerable volume of exudate (Naylor, 2002). In many instances, dressings will not cope adequately with this excess, and prolonged contact with the skin may occur.

In order to inform the clinician about the effects of specific treatment regimens on the skin surrounding a tumour, Grocott (1999) developed a scale to measure outcomes of care using TELER indicators (Le Roux, 1995; Grocott, 1999). TELER indicators were adapted to assist in measuring outcomes for the key variables of symptom control, dressing performance and the impact of the wound on patients with fungating lesions. *Table 2.2* lists the various categories of skin condition that may be associated with a fungating tumour.

Table 2.2: Skin condition indicator
0 = Skin is a diffuse fiery red with glazed appearance
1 = Skin is a diffuse fiery red
2 = Skin has fiery red patches
3 = Skin has patchy reddening
4 = Skin has pale pink patches
5 = Skin appears intact

Source: Grocott, 2000

Preventing excoriation and/or maceration of the peri-tumour skin from the action of exudate is an important aspect of care for two reasons: it promotes optimal levels of comfort for the patient while also ensuring that choice of dressing is not limited by poor condition of the peri-wound skin, eg. inability to apply adhesive dressing to excoriated skin.

Skin barrier preparations that contain alcohol are not recommended because of their potential to cause pain on application (Grocott, 2001). Grocott (2001) suggests two alternatives: a local anaesthetic gel containing lignocaine (Lutrol) and skin barrier preparations such as Cavilon™.

Another option is SuperSkin™, which appears to be an effective skin protectant (Hampton and Collins, 2001). This liquid barrier film provides a protective layer between the skin and any adhesive on dressings or tapes, while also assisting dressing or tape adhesion (Harding, 2002). It has similar properties to the adhesive used in Dermabond™ (Johnson & Johnson) and is based upon cyanoacrylate (superglue) (B Curtis, CliniMed, personal communication 2002). It provides protection from moisture and friction for up to three days by bonding directly to the skin. On application it has a no-sting effect as solvents or alcohols are not used. Another advantage of SuperSkin™ is its high MVTR, that allows the skin to breathe while still providing a barrier to water ingress (Harding, 2002).

Harding (2002) has presented some evaluative data indicating its usefulness as a skin protectant. Rolstad *et al* (1994) compared two prototype skin protectants — a siloxane-based polymer and an alcohol-based product — in the management of peri-wound skin in nineteen patients with a total of thirty wounds of varying aetiology. Results showed the siloxane-based polymer to be less painful on application and to produce greater improvement in skin condition than the alcohol-based product.

With regard to effective exudate management, Grocott (2001) believes there are 'significant limitations' with regard to the application of currently available dressings. A particular issue raised by Grocott (2001) is the lack of conformability of primary dressing to the fungating tumour. Grocott (2000) adds that, in general, optimal management in these situations is achieved through the following dressing capabilities: maintaining humidity; providing an absorptive capacity; and utilizing a high MVTR (to remove fluid in excess of that required for moist wound healing). It may also be relevant to consider the cosmetic capabilities of the dressing with regard to enhancing quality of life.

In an Australian study (postal questionnaire sent to specialist nurses in New South Wales) Wilkes *et al* (2001) found that alginates were the most popular choice of dressing in highly exuding, fungating wounds, followed by foams. Although the difficulty of managing heavy exudate in these wounds was raised, the issue of prevention or management of maceration was not overtly explored in this study.

Naylor (2002) recommends that where exudate levels are low, desiccation should be avoided by the use of low-absorbency products, eg. hydrocolloids or semi-permeable films. When exudate levels are moderate to high, hydro-polymer foam (Naylor, 2001), alginates, and hydrofibre are suitable, as are low-adherent dressings, such as soft silicone or knitted viscose, both used with a secondary absorbent pad. Naylor (2002) adds that for wounds with a small opening but high fluid output, a stoma appliance may be used.

Incontinence

Wound fluid is not the only cause of maceration: other sources of moisture may be implicated in its formation (Cutting and White, 2002a). The risk of developing pressure ulcers or other problems with the skin increases where there is incontinence, and faecal or urinary sources may result in maceration of the skin (Cutting and White, 2002a).

Protection of the skin is paramount if incontinence-related morbidity is to be avoided. For patients who have not responded to bladder/bowel training programmes, the application of disposable pads or absorbent disposable pants would appear to be the main approaches to management (Jeter and Lutz, 1996). Regular changing of the pads every two to three hours, with supplementary skin cleansing, application of moisturizer, barrier cream or skin protectant, augments this method of care (Jeter and Lutz, 1996).

Regular inspection of the skin, and taking care to avoid skin injury from friction and/or shear by correct utilization of positioning, turning, and transfer techniques, will avoid creating or extending skin damage. Barrier products such as SuperSkin™ or Cavilon™, which provide skin protection from faecal or urinary incontinence, should prove to be beneficial in these circumstances.

Intertrigo

Intertrigo is a cutaneous lesion arising from infection with *Candida albicans* (McMahon, 1994). It occurs between large skinfolds in obese patients, typically submammary, and presents as a wet, glazed, reddened lesion. McMahon (1994) evaluated a variety of treatments on sub-mammary intertrigo in a comparative study, and found thin hydrocolloid to be useful.

In this disorder, as with all relating to excess moisture and maceration, prevention is better than cure. Regular and detailed skin assessment of those at risk will help prevent the development of the problem.

Leg ulcers: arterial/ischaemic

Eschar may cover the wound bed of arterial ulcers. When the wound bed is visible it is regularly pale in colour and not the preferred pink/red of a healthy wound. The poor blood supply (ischaemia) is unlikely to generate a volume of wound fluid and consequently there is minimal exudate (Miller, 1999). Maceration therefore tends not to be a common problem in these wounds.

Leg ulcers: venous/mixed

The objectives of wound management for these ulcers include the need to 'maintain a moist wound environment without causing maceration' (Cullum, 1994).

Venous and complex or 'mixed' aetiology leg ulcers are usually exuding, even in the absence of frank infection (Wysocki *et al*, 1994). It is a challenge for the healthcare professional to utilize this moisture to the best effect. The wound bed should be kept at optimal or near-optimal level of moistness without excess, and the surrounding skin should be protected from the potentially damaging effects of exudate (Cutting and White, 2002b).

In a study designed to investigate the effects of occlusion on exudate generation in venous leg ulcers, Thomas *et al* (1996) attempted to correlate levels of exudate estimated subjectively by experienced nurses with levels measured quantitatively by absorption and weighing. Findings revealed that even experienced nurses were inconsistent in estimating exudate levels. The use of an adhesive, occlusive dressing (a hydrocolloid) was found to 'reduce' exudate generation, presumably by a negative feedback pressure mechanism.

Clinical research trials have shown a hydropolymer dressing to be effective in controlling exudate and avoiding maceration (Thomas *et al*, 1997; Taylor *et al*, 1999; Schulze *et al*, 2001).

In a comparative study on one hundred patients with venous leg ulcers, Thomas (1997) found that more ulcers treated with hydropolymer than those treated with the hydrocolloid comparator reduced in area (44/49 *vs* 34/47; *P*=0.028). There were more reports of leakage in the hydrocolloid group (27/50 *vs* 7/49; *P*=0.0001) and no reports of maceration in the hydropolymer group.

In a multicentre non-comparative study using a hydropolymer dressing, Taylor *et al* (1999) found very little leakage and only one case of recurrent maceration. Similarly, in a study on 113 patients with exuding leg ulcers randomized to alginate or hydropolymer (Schulze *et al*, 2001), maceration rates were lower in the hydropolymer group than in the alginate/film group. In this study, wear time was longer in the hydropolymer group (*P*=0.001). The combination of longer wear time with efficient exudate handling would be a cost-effective outcome, provided that the incidence of maceration is not increased (Trueman and Boothman, 2003). Recently, hydrocapillary dressings have also been demonstrated as safe and effective in managing exudate in venous leg ulcers (Karlsmark *et al*, 2004).

Lymphoedema

Lymphoedema occurs as a result of increased pressure within the lymphatic system due to either an increase in the volume of lymph or an alteration within the lymphatic vascular network, eg. blockage of a major vessel (Board and Harlow, 2003). During the initial stages of lymphoedema, it is unlikely that wound formation will be precipitated by this increase in pressure. Fluid may be seen on the skin surface without a wound being formed. Individuals with lymphoedema should take extra care to avoid traumatic damage to the skin. A wound exuding lymph is protein rich and therefore provides a ready medium for bacterial proliferation.

Skin changes may occur in chronic lymphoedema, with the development of hyperkeratosis, dry skin and callosities (Veitch, 1993). Cracks and fissures may form and fungal infections of the skin may develop, leading to secondary bacterial infection (Board and Harlow, 2003). Lymphorrhoea occurs when a large volume of lymph leaks on to the skin surface (Board and Harlow, 2002). In either situation — infection or lymphorrhoea — maceration may occur. Management should include appropriate absorbent dressings, emollients as a barrier agent, and antifungal agents or antibiotics for infection (Board and Harlow, 2002).

Neonatal wounds

The skin of the neonate is particularly fragile and liable to breakdown if the relevant conditions prevail. Children may succumb to a variety of wounds. Bale and Jones (1996) illustrate a number of causes of wounds in children, including extravasation injury, surgery, trauma (eg. abrasions, animal bites) and pressure ulcers. In a care report of a newborn infant, Irving (1999) suggests criteria that could be applied when choosing a suitable wound dressing. The dressing should: be sterile; take into account the size of the wound; not cause additional damage to the skin on removal; and be able to be left in place for a reasonable length of time.

Nappies, especially those with a plastic cover, may also cause maceration. They can create an environment that will induce maceration, particularly if left unchanged for long periods (McMahon, 1994). In these circumstances the skin of the infant is exposed to the water content of urine and faeces.

Additional causes of maceration in neonates include intertrigo (moisture and friction in opposed skin surfaces). This is more likely to occur in obese infants and may lead to secondary bacterial and fungal infections (McMahon, 1994).

Percutaneous enterostomal gastrostomy (PEG) sites

Although PEG sites may not be widely recognized as a wound in the classic sense, they do share many features with wounds (*Table 2.3*). The literature contains very little on how to recognize and manage the problem. Leak (2002) has reported local experience with problem PEG sites and offers an effective treatment option. In this and similar indications, eg. shunts, catheters and tracheostomies, there is a need to prevent maceration in the early stages as this should, in theory, reduce the development of hypergranulation and infection (Leak, 2003). Consequently, the use of absorbent dressings next to the skin should be considered when the patient is at risk of skin exposure to exudate and hence maceration. There is no evidence that the use of skin barrier preparations are of value.

Table 2.3: Features of PEG sites that are common to wounds

They are breaches in the dermis that do not heal (while the tube is *in situ*)

They are prone to exude and macerate

Overgranulation is common

They frequently become infected

Management of PEG site problems often falls to the responsibility of the wound care specialist nurse (and endoscopy nurses)

Problem PEG sites can adversely influence patient quality of life

PEG = percutaneous enterostomal gastrostomy

Pressure ulcers

'Pressure ulcer' appears to be the preferred term in the UK for lesions forming as a result of shear, friction or pressure in those with reduced mobility (Clark, 2004). Alternative nomenclature includes decubitus ulcers, bedsores or dermal ulcers. Cutting and White (2002a) have indicated that maceration may not only result from a wound but also be the cause. This latter form of maceration is particularly relevant to pressure ulcer development, where urinary incontinence, excessive sweating or water lost through the skin by transepidermal water loss (TEWL) may lead to skin breakdown. Whatever the cause, humidity and associated skin/wound temperature should be avoided so that conditions that will increase the likelihood of skin damage through maceration are not generated.

Careful management of the skin through the use of skin barrier products, moisturizers, absorbent pads and regular skin cleansing can ensure that the skin does not become macerated. If absorbent pads and/or underpants are used, it is preferable for them to have the capacity to wick any moisture away and not leave it in contact with the skin. It is crucial not to exceed appropriate wear time if this facility is to be used effectively.

Mechanical assaults on the skin (friction) may be avoided or reduced through careful patient-handling techniques and the application of suitable dressings, ie. ones that not only provide a barrier but also have a low friction coefficient with the surface with which they are in contact. Some transparent films and composite dressings have these properties but at varying levels.

Merck & Co Inc (2002) suggest that synthetic sheepskins may be of benefit in the prophylaxis of pressure ulcers. However, neither Marchand and Lidowski (1990) nor Watson (1990) recommend this approach for the management of patients at high risk of pressure ulcer development, although Dunford (1999) claims advantages when using 'natural' Australian Medical Sheepskins in vulnerable patients.

The National Pressure Ulcer Advisory Panel (NPUAP, 1992) suggests that maintaining humidity and temperature at levels that diminish skin problems, such as maceration, is the desired principle.

In clinical research, Thomas *et al* (1997) compared a hydropolymer with a hydrocolloid in ninety-nine patients with pressure ulcers treated in the community. The two groups were well matched for ulcer grade, duration and location. Results showed that the two groups had similar wear times and healing rates, but maceration was lower in the hydropolymer group (0/50 *vs* 4/49).

Radiation

Although rare, radiation damage to the skin, such as might occur after radiotherapy, gives rise to erythema and possible skin breakdown (Bennett and Moody, 1995c). Treatment is palliative as there is no means of reversing the damage (Hopewell, 1990). Skin erosions arising from laser damage can exude transiently but will heal (Haedersdal, 1999). Soft silicone dressings have been shown to be of value in this indication (Adamietz *et al*, 1995).

Skin sinuses

When exudate levels are particularly high and unrelenting, it is possible that the 'wound' is a discharging sinus. This is a track that extends from the skin surface to an underlying cavity, often an abscess. The track may be granulating, non-healing, malodorous, infected — all characteristics of a typical wound.

Detailed sinus management guidelines have been reported by Butcher (1999). He recommends a thorough examination of the sinus and surrounding area, as well as the exudate (volume, colour and consistency). All sinuses should be swabbed for culture and sensitivity testing. The dressing (conservative) management should prevent premature closure (which would lead to a painful extension of the underlying cavity) and be able to cope with exudate. This entails the frequent use of absorbent materials in ribbon or rope form, eg. alginates and hydrofibre, with secondary dressings, such as hydropolymer or hydrocolloid. According to Butcher (1999), the dressing must facilitate free drainage of exudate, be pain-free in application and removal, control and absorb exudate, and protect the surrounding skin. A barrier skin preparation may be useful in this latter respect.

Surgical wounds

Surgical wounds closed by suture generally heal rapidly as they have been imposed on healthy tissue (Watret and White, 2001) without the impediments of an underlying pathology or an imposing bacterial burden. Consequently, it is rare for them to succumb to maceration as the conditions that would encourage its development are not present.

Criteria for the 'ideal' surgical wound dressing have been proposed by Watret and White (2001). Dry dressings are widely used on wounds healing by first intention, but these run the risk of adhering to the wound and thus causing pain and trauma on removal (Bennett and Moody, 1995b; Collier and Hollinworth, 2000).

If the wound is left to heal through secondary intention the volume of exudate will be somewhat dependent on the size and depth of the wound (Harding *et al*, 1986), ie. the bigger the wound the more exudate it is likely to produce. Increased volume of exudate may put the wound at risk of maceration if it is not managed correctly. Accurate assessment is vital if optimal management is to be achieved. Ongoing evaluation will also be required to accommodate the dynamic process of wound repair.

The desire to disturb the wound as little as possible so as not to disrupt the repair process unnecessarily may lead to dressings being left *in situ* for unreasonable lengths of time, causing maceration.

Additionally, prolonged wear time, notably to seven days, is often promoted by medical device companies in an effort to establish cost-effectiveness of their products. The result is unrealistic wear time which may lead to maceration as all dressings have a finite capacity to handle large volumes of exudate.

Conclusions

It is no longer appropriate, for the goal of achieving healing, to use dressings that simply absorb and remove exudate while still maintaining a moist environment. Knowledge of wound exudate, combined with assessment guidelines, enable the clinician to practice from an informed perspective when managing exuding wounds. The vast choice of primary and secondary dressings available permits the practitioner, with judicious selection, to achieve an 'optimal' moist environment. This must be the management goal for each of the range of exuding wound types if maceration is to be avoided and healing optimized.

> ## Key points
>
> ⌘ Dressings have a role to play in the prevention and management of maceration.
>
> ⌘ Before a dressing regimen is considered, the root cause must be assessed.
>
> ⌘ Skin protection is vital.
>
> ⌘ Different wound types have varying requirements for managment.
>
> ⌘ It is important for the practitioner to have a thorough understanding of the nature and causes of wound exudate.

References

Adamietz IA, Mose AS, Haberl A, Saran FH, Thilmann C, Bottcher HD (1995) Effect of self-adhesive, silicone-coated polyamide net dressing on irradiated human skin. *Radiation Oncology Investigations* **2**: 277–82

Alexander JW, Fischer JE, Morris MJ (1983) The influence of hair removal on wound infections. *Arch Surg* **118**: 347–52

Attwood AI (1989) Calcium alginate dressing accelerates graft donor site healing. *J Plast Surg* **43**: 373–79

Bale S, Jones V (1996) Caring for children with wounds. *J Wound Care* **5**(4): 177–180

Bennett G, Moody M, eds (1995a) Principles of wound management. In: *Wound Care for Health Professionals*. Chapman & Hall, London: 49–66

Bennett G, Moody M (1995b) The holistic approach to wound assessment. In: *Wound Care for Health Professionals*. Chapman & Hall, London: 34–47

Bennett G, Moody M, eds (1995c) Management of complex and difficult-to-heal wounds. In: *Wound Care for Health Professionals*. Chapman & Hall, London: 130–1

Bishop SM, Walker M, Rogers A, Chen WYJ (2003) Importance of moisture balance at the wound-dressing interface. *J Wound Care* **12**(4): 125–8

Board J, Harlow W (2002) Lymphoedema 3: the available treatments for lymphoedema. *Br J Nurs* **11**(7): 438–50

Board J, Harlow W (2003) Lymphoedema. In: White RJ, eds. *Trends in Wound Care, volume II*. Quay Books, Dinton, Salisbury: 62–72

Brady SC, Snelling CF, Chow G (1980) Comparison of donor site dressings. *Ann Plast Surg* **5**: 238–43

Brotherston TM, Lawrence JC (1993) Dressings for donor sites. *J Wound Care* **2**: 84–8

Burch J (2004) The management and care of people with stoma complications. *Br J Nurs* **13**(6): 307–18

Burns DA (1998) Skin infections. In: Monk BE, Graham-Brown R, Sarkany I, eds. *Skin Disorders in the Elderly*. Blackwell Scientific Publications, Oxford

Butcher M (1999) Management of wound sinuses. *J Wound Care* **8**: 451–4

Cameron J (1998) Skin care for patients with chronic leg ulcers. *J Wound Care* **7**: 459–62

Cameron J, Newton H (2003) *Skin Care in Wound Management*. IWM Educational Booklet, Medical Communications Ltd, Holsworthy

Cameron J, Hofman D, Wilson JM, Powell SM, Cherry GW (2003) A comparison of two peri-wound skin protectants in venous leg ulcers: a randomized controlled trial. Poster presentation to the Society of American Wound Care (SAWC), Las Vegas, USA, April 2003

Clark M (2004) Models of pressure ulcer care: costs and outcome. In: Clark M, ed. *Pressure Ulcers: Recent advances in tissue viability*. Quay Books, MA Healthcare Limited, Dinton, Salisbury

Collier M (2003) The challenge of wound exudate. *Nurs Times* **99**(5): 47–8

Collier M, Hollinworth H (2000) Pain and tissue trauma during dressing change. *Nurs Stand* **14**(40): 71–3

Cullum N (1994) Leg ulcer treatments: a critical review (part 1). *Nurs Stand* **9**(1): 29–33

Cutting KF (1999) The causes and prevention of maceration of the skin. *J Wound Care* **8**(4): 200–1

Cutting KF, White RJ (2002a) Maceration of the skin: 1: the nature and causes of skin maceration. *J Wound Care* **11**(7): 275–8

Cutting KF, White RJ (2002b) Avoidance and management of peri-wound skin maceration. *Prof Nurse* **18**(1): 33–6

Dunford C (1999) Down-under wool. Sheepskins and Medi-Wool. Online at: http://www.medicalsheepskins.com/ testimonials.htm (accessed 28.10.03)

Dykes PJ, Heggie R (2001) Effects of adhesive dressings on the stratum corneum of the skin. *J Wound Care* **10**(1): 7–10

Dykes PJ, Heggie R (2003) The link between the peel force of adhesive dressings and subjective discomfort in volunteer subjects. *J Wound Care* **12**(7): 260–2

Edwards R, Harding KG (2004) Bacteria and wound healing. *Curr Opin Infect Dis* **17**(2): 91–6

Flanagan M (1996) A practical framework for wound assessment. 1: physiology. *Br J Nurs* **5**(22): 1391–7

Feldman DL (1991) Which dressing for split-thickness skin graft donor sites? *Ann Plast Surg* **27**: 288–91

Fletcher J (2003) Managing wound exudate. *Nurs Times* **99**(5): 51–2

Fowler A, Dempsey A (1998) Split-thickness skin graft donor sites. *J Wound Care* **7**(8): 399–402

Gray D, White RJ (2004) The wound exudate continuum. *Applied Wound Management* (Suppl) **1**(1): 19–22, Wounds-UK, Aberdeen

Grocott P (1999) An evaluation of the palliative management of fungating malignant wounds within a multiple case study design. PhD thesis, King's College University London

Grocott P (2000) The palliative management of fungating malignant wounds. *J Wound Care* **9**(1): 4–9

Grocott P (2001) The palliative management of fungating malignant wounds. In: Hollingworth H, ed. *Wound Care Society Educational Booklet*. Wound Care Society, Huntingdon

Haedersdal M (1999) Cutaneous side-effects from laser treatment of the skin. *Acta Derm Venereol (Stockh)* Suppl **207**: 1–32

Harding KG, Hughes LE, Marks J (1986) *A Guide to the Practical Management of Granulating Wounds*. Valbonne Cedex, Dow Corning

Harding N (2002) A practice-based evaluation of a liquid barrier film. *Int J Palliat Nurs* **8**(5): 233–4, 236–9

Hampton S, Collins F (2001) SuperSkin: the management of skin susceptible to breakdown. *Br J Nurs* **10**(11): 742–6

Hopewell J W (1990) The skin: its structure and response to ionizing radiation. *Int J Radiat Biol* **57**(4): 751–73

Imokawa G (2001) Lipid abnormalities in atopic dermatitis. *J Am Acad Dermatol* **45**(Suppl): S29–S32

Irving V (1999) Management of a neonatal wound on a newborn infant. *J Wound Care* **8**(10): 485–86

Jakobsson O, Bjorklund C (2000) A treatment for split-skin donor sites. In: *Aquacel: New Dimensions in the Treatment of Post-surgical Wounds*. Proceedings of a satellite symposium, EWMA, Stockholm, May 2000. Medical Communications, Holsworthy, UK

James JH, Watson ACH (1975) The use of Opsite, a vapour-permeable dressing, on skin graft donor sites. *J Plast Surg* **28**: 107–10

Jeter KF, Lutz JB (1996) Skin care in the frail elderly dependent incontinent patient. *Adv Wound Care* **9**(1): 29–34

Jones V (2004) Wound bed preparation and its implications for practice. *Applied Wound Management* (Suppl) **1**(1): 4–9. Wounds-UK, Aberdeen

Karlsmark T, Hahn TW, Thomsen JK, Gottrup F (2004) Hydrocapillary dressing to manage exudate in venous leg ulcers. *Br J Nurs* (Suppl) **13**(6): S29–S35

Kingsley A, White RJ, Gray D (2004) The wound infection continuum. *Applied Wound Management* (Suppl) **1**(1): 13–19. Wounds-UK, Aberdeen

Lamke L, Nilsson GE, Reithner HL (1997) The evaporative water loss from burns and water permeability of grafts and artificial membranes used in the treatment of burns. *Burns* **3**: 159–65

Le Roux AA (1995) TELER: the concept. *Physiotherapy* **79**(11): 755–8

Leak K (2002) PEG site infections: a novel use for Actisorb Silver 220. *Br J Community Nurs* **7**(6): 321–5

Leak K (2003) Changing wound care practice: management of PEG sites. In: White RJ, ed. *The Silver Book*. Quay Books, MA Healthcare Limited, Dinton, Salisbury

Leung DYM, Bieber T (2003) Atopic dermatitis. *Lancet* **361:** 151–60

McMahon R (1994) Evaluation of topical nursing interventions in the treatment of sub-mammary lesions. In: *Proceedings of the 4th EWMA Conference on Advances in Wound Management*. Harrogate, UK

Marchand AC, Lidowski H (1990) Reassessment of the use of genuine sheepskin for pressure ulcer prevention and treatment. *Decubitus* **6**(1): 44–7

MEDLINEplus (2002) Online at: http://www2.merriam-webster.com/cgi-bin/mwmednlm?book= Medical&va=wound (accessed 5 November 2003)

Merck & Co Inc (2002) *The Merck Manual of Diagnosis and Therapy*. Chapter 122. Online at: http://www.merck.com/pubs/mmanual/section10/chapter122/122a.htm (accessed 3.11.03)

Metcalf C (1999) Enterocutaneous fistulae. *J Wound Care* **8**(3): 141–2

Miller M (1999) Wound assessment. In: Miller M, Glover D, eds. *Wound Management Theory and Practice*. Nursing Times Books, London: 23–36

Naylor W (2001) Using a new foam dressing in the care of fungating wounds. *Br J Nurs* **10**(6): Suppl S24–S31

Naylor W (2002) Part 1: Symptom control in the management of fungating wounds. World Wide Wounds. Online at: http://www.worldwidewounds.com/ 2002/march/Naylor/Symptom-Control Fungating-Wounds.html (accessed 28.10.03)

Newton H, Cameron J (2003) *Skin Care in Wound Management*. IWM Educational Book, Medical Communications (UK) Ltd, Holsworthy

NPUAP (1992) *Statement on Pressure Ulcer Prevention 1992*. NPUAP, Reston Virginia. Online at: http://www.npuap.org/positn1.htm (accessed 28.10.03)

Orth DS (1993) *Handbook of Cosmetic Microbiology*. Marcel Dekker, New York: 1–18

Palamand S, Reed AM, Weimann LJ (1992) Testing intelligent wound dressings. *J Biomater Appl* **6**(3): 198–215

Rolstad BS, Borchert K, Magnam S, Scheel N (1994) An observational comparison study to evaluate an alcohol-based and a siloxane-based skin protectant in the management of peri-wound skin. In: Harding KG, Dealey C, Cherry G, Gottrup F, eds. *Proceedings of the 3rd European Conference on Advances in Wound Management*. Harrogate, UK. Macmillan Magazines Ltd, London

Rottmann WL, Grove G, Lutz JB, Burton SA, Rolstad BS (1993) Scientific basis of protecting peri-wound skin. In: Harding KG, Dealey C, Cherry G, Gottrup F, eds. *Proceedings of the 3rd European Conference on Advances in Wound Management*. Harrogate, UK. Macmillan Magazines Ltd, London

Schulze H-J, Lane C, Charles H, Ballard K, Hampton S, Moll I (2001) Evaluating a superabsorbent hydropolymer dressing for exuding venous ulcers. *J Wound Care* **10**(1): 511–17

Springett K, White RJ (2003) Skin changes in the at-risk foot. In: White RJ, ed. *Trends in Wound Care, volume II*. Quay Books, MA Healthcare Limited, Dinton, Salisbury

Taylor A, Lane C, Walsh J, Young S (1999) A non-comparative multi-centre clinical evaluation of a new hydropolymer dressing. *J Wound Care* **8**(9): 489–92

Thomas S (1992) Alginates. *J Wound Care* **1**(1): 29–32

Thomas S (1997) Assessment and management of wound exudate. *J Wound Care* **6**(7): 327–30

Thomas S (1998) The importance of secondary dressings in wound care. *J Wound Care* **7**(4): 189–92

Thomas S, Fear M, Humphreys J, Disley L, Waring M (1996) The effect of dressings on the production of exudate from venous leg ulcers. *Wounds* **8**(5): 145–50

Thomas S, Banks V, Bales S, Fear-Price M, Harding KG (1997) A comparison of two dressings in the management of chronic wounds. *J Wound Care* **6**(8): 383–6

Trueman P, Boothman S (2003) Tielle Plus fluid handling capacity can lead to cost savings. *Br J Nurs* **12**(16): Suppl 18–22

Veitch J (1993) Skin problems in lymphoedema. *Wound Manage* **4**(2): 42–5

Vowden K, Vowden P (2003) Wound Bed Preparation. World Wide Wounds (http://www.worldwidewounds.com/2002/april/Vowden/Wound-Bed-Preparation.html) (accessed 4 November 2003)

Watret L, White R (2001) Surgical wound management: the role of dressings. *Nurs Stand* **15**(44): 59–69

Watson R (1990) How effective are sheepskins? *Nursing Elderly* **Sept/Oct:** 14–15

White R (2001) Managing exudate. *Nurs Times* **97**(14): 59–60

White RJ, Cutting KF (2003) Interventions to avoid maceration of the skin and wound bed. *Br J Nurs* **12**(20): 1186–1201

White RJ, Dods IA, Vickers CFH (1990) A study of the epidermal barrier in atopic dermatitis. In: Czernielewski JM, ed. *Immunological and Pharmacological Aspects of Atopic and Contact Eczema.* Karger, Basel: 194–7

Wilkes L, White K, Smeal T, Beale B (2001) Malignant wound management: what dressings do nurses use? *J Wound Care* **10**(3): 65–9

Wysocki AB, Staiano-Coico L, Grinnell F (1994) Wound fluid from chronic leg ulcers. *J Invest Dermatol* **101:** 64–68

3

Exudate: Composition and functions

Keith F Cutting

Wound exudate is all too often perceived as a clinical management problem. While this can be the case, it should be recognized that exudate does fulfil an important function in the healing process. Gradual acceptance of the benefits of moist wound healing, combined with the current goals of the 'ideal' moist environment, focuses attention on the role of exudate. This chapter is intended to define the components and functions of 'normal' exudate and, by comparison, differentiate abnormal exudate.

The presence of exudate influences the process of wound healing and the patient's quality of life, but it is not aesthetically pleasing for either the clinician or the patient. Consequently, it is important to manage exudate, typically by the use of selected dressings, in an attempt to provide an optimum moist wound environment, and, to mask the unpleasant visual and odour aspects.

If wounds produce exudate at regular, insignificant, levels then the need for habitual change of dressing would be similarly infrequent. In this unlikely event we could become distracted from the need to examine exudate and to understand what it is composed of and the role it has to play in the healing process.

Defining exudate

In terms of assessment, exudate can provide information on the status of the wound. It can help in the diagnosis of infection (volume, consistency, colour), it assists in monitoring healing and judgements can be made on the choice of topical applications. A healthy wound will generate a small level of moisture that will be apparent on its surface.

As yet, the optimal level of exudate required to facilitate the healing process is undetermined and this varies with different types of wound. Exudate volume is traditionally categorised as light, moderate or heavy, but this approach is subjective and leads to problems with dressing selection (Thomas *et al*, 1996). An attempt has been made to improve on this situation (Bates-Jensen, 1997) by developing a number of descriptors (*Table 3.1*) that are more detailed than those mentioned above. By reducing subjective elements and assessing exudate volume, through the use of a measuring guide, offers the clinician an opportunity to improve on estimated volume accuracy.

Different types of wounds in varying conditions express various types of exudate. Bates-Jensen (1997) illustrates different exudate types that may be encountered (*Table 3.2*).

Table 3.1: Exudate descriptors by volume		
None	=	wounds tissues dry
Scant	=	wound tissues moist
Small	=	wound tissues wet; moisture evenly distributed in wound; drainage involves 25% of dressing
Moderate	=	wound tissues saturated; drainage may or may not be evenly distributed in wound; drainage involves 25% to 75% of dressing
Large	=	wound tissues bathed in fluid; drainage freely expressed; may or may not be evenly distributed in wound; drainage involves 75% of dressing

Table 3.2: Types of exudate		
Bloody	=	thin, bright, watery
Serosanguinous	=	thin, watery. pale red to pink
Serous	=	thin, watery, clear
Purulent	=	thin or thick, opaque tan to yellow
Foul purulent	=	thick, opaque yellow to green with offensive odour

Despite the assistance rendered from using the above developments, the difficulties persist in assessing exudate volume irrespective of the type of exudate generated. Thomas *et al* (1996) have clearly demonstrated this even when experienced nurses were involved in an assessment of exudate levels in venous leg ulcers. He found that even such experienced practitioners were unable to agree on exudate levels.

The term exudate is a generic one used to identify liquid produced from wounds (Thomas, 1997). A simple answer to the question 'what is it?' could include Paracelsus' (1493–1541) statement that it is nature's balsam (Haeger, 1989). This might appear to be a simplistic approach in our quest for a clear understanding of exudate. However, if the definition of balsam as a healing agent is accepted then Paracelsus' observation appears to take on a greater degree of relevance.

Exudate is generated as part of the inflammatory response (White and Hothersall, 2002; White, 2001). It is essential to the healing process and, together with inflammation, should not be considered as a necessary evil but as a vital component of the reparative process.

In wounds healing through primary intention a small amount of exudate will be viewed on the apposed edges of the skin providing an effective seal to bacteria and debris. A narrow border of erythema will surround the incised edges and together with the dried surface exudate is a normal and welcome sign that healing is progressing.

Despite the advances made in wound care, our knowledge of exudate remains somewhat rudimentary. The intention here is to provide an overview of exudate in respect of its composition and function.

'Normal' (serous) exudate has a high protein content with a specific gravity greater than 1.020. It contains essential nutrients for epithelial cells, facilitates the ingress of white cells and provides the moist environment so important for healing. It also contains electrolytes and a number of inflammatory components, such as leukocytes, fibrinogen and fibrin.

In the unwounded state, the dermal cells are kept moist by the protective epidermis (Thomas, 1997). However, when a wound occurs, moisture (exudate) present on the wound surface prevents desiccation that may lead to delayed healing (Hinman and Maibach, 1963).

The volume of exudate (fluid, liquid, drainage) that exudes from a wound is most prominent during the inflammatory and proliferative stages of the healing process. The volume produced will vary not only at different stages of the healing continuum but will alter between different wound types depending on their origin and location and in relation to wound size.

Just as the healing process is a dynamic one, so too is exudate content. The contribution that exudate makes to the healing process can be seen from analysis of acute wound fluid (AWF) (*Figure 3.1*). Here, the analogy of exudate as a healing agent appears to be more appropriate than when applied to chronic wounds. A healthy wound contains endogenous protein degrading enzymes, known as proteases or proteinases. These include serine proteinase, cysteine proteinase, aspartic proteinase and matrix metalloproteinases (MMPs) (Falanga, 2002).

The role of these endogenous proteinases is to assist in preparation of the wound bed and to degrade components of the extracellular matrix, eg. collagens and elastin, prior to wound closure and remodelling. Moist wound healing is advocated as the preferred approach to healing not just because of the advantages to the rate of epithelialisation (Winter, 1962) but because slough (dead protein) is often removed efficiently through the process of autolysis. This is because endogenous proteinases are active de-sloughing agents and are delivered to the wound bed via exudate that is produced as part of the inflammatory reaction. Differences exist between the levels of MMPs, TIMPS and cytokines found in exudate in acute and chronic wounds (Baker and Leaper, 2000). Additionally, membrane bound proteinases have a valuable role to play in healing by allowing keratinocytes and endothelial cells to forge a trail as they migrate through tissue (Saarialho-Kere, 1998). The activity of these degrading enzymes are controlled by tissue inhibitors of metalloproteinases (TIMPs). TIMPs are a group of related proteins that not only inhibit MMP activity but also have positive effects on cell growth (Thomas, 2001).

Neutrophils (initial infiltrate of predominantly inflammatory cells) are attracted to the wound site by a variety of chemotactic agents. They arrive via the blood stream and are additionally transported in extravasated plasma to the wound bed. Neutrophils commence the wound cleansing process preceding macrophage and protease activity. They migrate to the wounded tissue almost immediately following injury and through phagocytic activity commence removal of debris, bacteria and devitalised tissue. In addition, they release further inflammatory mediators.

Phagocytic monocytes are attracted to the wound site and after a few days they differentiate into macrophages. These cells are considered fundamental to the repair process (Clark, 1985). Macrophages continue with wound cleansing by phagocytosis of bacteria and debris, and by producing elastase and collagenase, thus contribute to the process of autolysis.

Sodium Potassium Chloride Urea Creatinine }	similar concentrations to that found in serum (Vickery 1997)
Glucose	lower levels compared to blood (Randolph May, 1982) probably due to neutrophil utilisation
Cytokines	Acute wound fluid is enriched with growth factors (Chen, 1998). IL1-ß, IL-6, IL-8, TNF-α, Interferon α found in mastectomy wound fluid (Vickery, 1997). IL-6, IL-1ß and TNF-α levels higher in colorectal wound fluid when compared with breast fluid (Baker and Leaper 2000).
Leucocytes	Initially similar levels to whole blood but differential counts change within a few hours of wounding (Vickery 1997)
Lysozyme	Elevated levels compared to serum found in donor site fluid (Buchan *et al*, 1980).
Macrophages	Significant numbers appear three to five days post wounding (Vickery, 1997).
Metalloproteinases	MMPs present but in inactive pre-enzyme stage (Wysocki *et al*, 1993). MMP2, MMP9 — levels rise post wounding but fall to baseline levels within forty-eight hours (Vickery, 1997). Differences detected in MMP and TIMP expression between mastectomy and colorectal surgery samples but no significant difference in total MMP activity (Baker and Leaper, 2000).
Micro-organisms	Presence of micro-organisms does not necessarily imply infection. Acute wounds likely colonised by aerobes (Bowler and Davies, 1999).
Neutrophils	The predominant white cell three to four hours post wounding (Vickery, 1997)
Protein	Lower levels than serum (Vickery, 1997)

Figure 3.1: Acute wound fluid — constituents

Some differences between acute and chronic wound fluid may be seen in *Table 3.3* below.

Table 3.3: Some differences between acute and chronic wound fluid	
Acute	**Chronic**
Fluid supports cell proliferation	Fluid does not support cell proliferation
Fluid does not damage peri-wound skin	Fluid damages peri-wound skin
Fibronectin intact Neutrophil elastase, serine and MMP levels normal	Fibronectin degraded neutrophil elastase, serin and MMP levels high
Fibroblast mitosis present	Fibroblast mitosis altered

Exudate may be regarded as a transport mechanism. Plasma, from which exudate is derived, delivers all the necessary ingredients, oxygen and nutrients, to the tissues and organs of the body. Similarly, exudate on its way to the surface delivers these components to the wound bed.

In the acute wound the volume of exudate is usually of manageable proportions, whereas in chronic wounds the situation may be less predictable. The volume and type of exudate varies depending on the prevailing circumstances. Despite the problems that may be generated by chronic wound exudate, such as enzymatic degradation of exposed healthy skin or wound bed and exudate-mediated maceration, clinicians do not normally advocate total removal or elimination of exudate. It is not just the aqueous component that may positively influence healing, but also the solutes. The trend for generating an optimal moist environment generally focuses more on managing exudate rather than seeking its complete removal, even though Chen (1998) has described chronic wound exudate as a wounding agent in its own right. Conversely, a decrease in exudate production is usually interpreted as a positive indication that healing is progressing.

Trengove *et al* (1996) showed that in healing wounds, concentrations of glucose, bicarbonate and total protein increase. Additionally, concentrations of C-reactive protein, an inflammatory marker, decrease in exudate and in serum. James and Taylor (1997) have pointed out that C-reactive protein, which may be assayed from serum, (easier to collect than exudate) may have the potential to act as an indicator of the status of the wound.

Chronic wounds are a result of chronic inflammation. This is characterised by a cycle of cellular activity that does not support healing. Chronic wound exudate contains active degrading enzymes and these have a vital role to play in the repair process; these lyse devitalised protein and debris and thus assist in preparing the wound for healing. However, this proteolytic activity can be inappropriate (ie. prolonged beyond the useful period) and so contribute to wound chronicity (Brantigan, 1996; Taylor and James, 2001; Moore, 2003). Matrix metalloprotease and serine protease levels are elevated when compared with acute wound fluid (Taylor and James, 2001). In chronic wounds that are progressing towards healing, lactate levels fall but albumin, total protein and glucose levels rise (Taylor and James, 2001).

Component	Function
Fibrin	Clotting
Platelets	Clotting
Polymorphonuclear cells (PMNs)	Immune defence, production of growth factors
Lymphocytes	Immune defence
Macrophages	Immune defence, production of growth factors
Microorganisms	Exogenous factor
Plasma proteins, albumin, globulin, fibrinogen	Maintain osmotic pressure, immunity, transport of macromolecules
Lactic acid	Product of cellular metabolism and indicating biochemical hypoxia (James *et al*, 1997)
Glucose	Cellular energy source
Inorganic salts	Buffering, pH hydrogen ion concentration in a solution
Growth factors	Proteins controlling factor specific healing activities
Wound debris/dead cells	No function
Proteolytic enzymes	Enzymes that degrade protein, including serine, cysteine, aspartic proteases and matrix metalloproteinases (MMPs)
TIMPS	Controlled inhibition of metalloproteinases

Figure 3.2: Some constituents of exudate and their function

Currently our knowledge relating to volume of exudate produced by different wounds is limited. Lamke and Nilsson (1997) have shown that burns produce in excess of 5000g/m²/day of exudate. In a study of ten venous leg ulcers, Thomas (1997) measured exudate production as ranging between 4000–12000g/m²/day. If exudate levels remain heavy this may be due to untreated underlying pathology (uncontrolled oedema) or an increasing bioburden that may progress to infection. In either situation healing will not be advanced until these issues are addressed. However, we have yet to gain a full understanding as to why some wounds produce more exudate than others. Exudate analysis may indicate protein loss that in some instances may be of clinical significance (Nelson, 1997).

The dynamic nature of wound exudate content is demonstrated if a wound becomes infected. Microorganisms may be considered to be exogenous components and their presence will often lead to an increase in exudate production (Gilchrist, 1999). An attempt to rationalise this phenomenon is offered by Neilsen *et al* (2001) and White and Hothersall (2002) who hypothesised that the release of bacterial exotoxins acting on vascular endothelial growth factor (VEGF) increases vascular permeability, and hence exudate production. It is likely that additional factors yet to be identified are implicated in enhancing vascular permeability.

Some bacterial species thrive in a moist environment. For example, two common wound pathogens flourish in a high water activity (aw) level — for example, *Staphylococcus aureus* has a_w 0.96 and *Pseudomonas aeruginosa* a_w 0.86. This raises the question: does wound fluid (maintaining a moist environment) increase the risk of bacterial infection? Hinman and Maibach (1963) generated initial concerns when they noticed that on desiccation bacteria died. Subsequent investigation has challenged this assumption and Hohn *et al* (1977) demonstrated that wound fluid suppressed bacterial growth. A number of other papers have supported this assertion, most notably a meta-analysis of infection rates under occlusive dressings which showed that infection was less likely to occur under occlusion (Hutchinson 1989). This beneficial effect is partly attributed to the fact that neutrophils thrive in a moist environment. Thus, it appears that exudate has a role to play in keeping a wound free of infection.

It is also interesting to note that levels of MMPs rise dramatically if the wound becomes infected; some bacterial virulence factors, known as invasins, are also MMPs (Cooper, 2003). As these proteases degrade extra-cellular matrix proteins, this may be considered an additional factor in regression of healing. This deterioration in the wound may also be detected before clinical signs of infection become apparent (Vickery, 1997). Additionally, acute wound fluid appears to support fibroblast mitotic activity (unlike chronic wound fluid) thereby indicating that the inflammatory mediators and cellular components of AWF actively support healing *Figure 3.1* and *Table 3.3* above help to illustrate this.

If a wound becomes infected the nature and volume of the exudate may change. For example, if the infection is due to the predominance of *Pseudomonas aeruginosa*, the exudate becomes thicker and green-blue in colour (Villavicencio, 1998). Other types of exudate (Cutting and White, 2002) may be seen below (*Figure 3.3*).

Serous:	Clear, watery consistency. Possibly a sign of infection. Some bacteria produce fibrinolysins, which degrade fibrin clots or coagulated plasma. Some strains of *Staphylococcus aureus*, ß-haemolytic group A streptococci, B. fragilis produce fibrinolysins and *Pseudomonas aeruginosa* produce a non-specific enzyme that degrades fibrin.
Fibrinous:	Cloudy, contains fibrin protein strands.
Purulent:	Pyogenic organisms and other inflammatory cells.
Haemo-purulent:	Contains neutrophils, dead/dying bacteria and inflammatory cells, ie. established infection is present. Consequent damage to dermal capillaries leads to blood leakage.
Haemorrhagic:	Capillaries have become so friable that they easily break down and spontaneous, copious bleeding occurs. Blood is the major component of this type of exudate. Do not confuse with bloody exudate from over enthusiastic debridement.

Figure 3.3: Nature of exudate

Exudate has the potential for providing a vast amount of information in respect of wound status. Biochemical analysis provides, as yet, limited information on wound bed cytokines, proteases and a number of biochemical markers. Quantitative and qualitative analysis of these agents currently provides some insight in respect of the progression/regression of a wound. A comprehensive analysis of wound bed exudate constituents is required if an informed judgement is to made. Further work is required to define/clarify the differences that exist in exudate composition of acute and chronic non-healing wounds. Similarly, more information on the composition of the microflora content of exudate requires further investigation, taking into account the effects and influences of bacterial synergy. Inferences, at this time, should be reserved on the presence or absence of infection when based on quantitative bacterial analysis.

Perhaps in time this information will support the development of therapies that will avoid the development of chronicity, or, enable those wounds that do become chronic to be transferred to an acute state where they may rapidly progress towards healing.

Key points

⌘　Production of exudate is a normal event.

⌘　Important differences exist between the exudates produced by acute and chronic wounds.

⌘　Exudate contains endogenous proteases that prepare the wound bed for healing.

⌘　Proteolytic activity in chronic wounds can be inappropriate (unregulated).

⌘　An increase in exudate levels may indicate a deteriorating wound.

References

Baker EA, Leaper DJ (2000) Proteinases, their inhibitors and cytokine profiles in acute wound fluid. *Wound Repair and Regeneration* **8**(5): 392–8

Bates-Jensen MB (1997) The pressure sore status tool — a few thousand assessments later. *Adv Wound Care* **10**(5): 65–73

Bowler PG, Davies BJ (1999) The microbiology of acute and chronic wounds. *Wounds* **11**(4):72–8

Buchan IA, Andrews JK, Lang SM (1980) Clinical and laboratory investigations of the composition and properties of human skin wound exudate under semi-permeable dressings. *Burns* **7**: 326–34

Brantigan CO (1996) The history of the understanding of growth factors in wound healing. *Wounds* **8**(3): 78–90

Chen J (1998) *Aquacel hydrofibre dressing: The next step in wound dressing technology*. Monograph. ConvaTec, London

Clark RAF (1985) Cutaneous tissue repair: basic biological considerations. *J Am Acad Dermatol* **13** :701–25

Cooper RA (2003) The contribution of microbial virulence to infection. In: White RJ, ed. *The Silver Book*. Quay Books, MA Healthcare Limited, Dinton, Salisbury

Cutting KF, White R (2002) Maceration of the skin and wound bed: 1; Its nature and causes. *J Wound Care* **11**(7): 275–8

Falanga V (2002) Wound bed preparation and the role of enzymes; a case for multiple actions of therapeutic agents. *Wounds* **14**(2): 47–57.

Gilchrist B (1999) Wound infection. In: Miller M, Glover D, eds. *Wound Management Theory and Practice*. EMAP Healthcare Ltd, London:100

Haeger K (1989) *The Illustrated History of Surgery*. Harold Starke, London

Hinman CD, Maibach H (1963) Effect on air exposure and occlusion on experimental human skin wounds. *Nature* **200**: 377–8

Hohn DC, Granelli SG, Burton RW, Hunt TK (1977) Antimicrobial systems of the surgical wound. II. Detection of antimicrobial protein in cell-free wound fluid. *Am J Surg* **133**(5): 601–6

Hutchinson JJ (1989) Prevalence of wound infection under occlusive dressings: a collective survey of reported research. *Wounds* **1**(2); 123–33

James T, Hughes M, Taylor R Cherry G (1997) Biochemical measurements in wound fluid In: Cherry G, Harding K, eds. Management of Wound Exudate: Abstracts from the first combined meeting of the European Tissue Repair Society and the European Wound Management Association at Green College University of Oxford. ETRS Bulletin

Lamke LO, Nilsson CE (1997) The evaporative water loss from burns and water vapour permeability of grafts and artificial membranes used in treatment of burns. *Burns* **3**:159–65

Moore K (2003) Compromised wound healing: a scientific approach to treatment. *Br J Comm Nurs* **8**(6): 274–8

Neilsen H J, Werther K, Mynster T *et al* (2001) Bacterial-induced release of white cell and platelet-derived vascular endothelial growth factor. *Vox Sang* **80**(3): 170–8

Nelson A (1997) Is exudate a clinical problem? In: Cherry G, Harding K, eds. Management of wound exudate. Joint meeting European Wound Management Association and European Tissue Repair Society, Green College Oxford. London, Churchill

Randolph MS (1982) Physiological activity from an occlusive wound dressing. In: Lawrence JC, ed. Proceedings of a Symposium, Queen Elizabeth Postgraduate Medical Centre, Birmingham, England. Oxford, Medical Publishing Foundation: 27-51

Saarialho-Kere UK (1998) Patterns of matrix metalloproteinase and TIMP expression in chronic ulcers. *Arch Dermatol Res* **290** Suppl: S47-54

Taylor R, James T (2001) Wound fluid: an indicator of wound bed status. In: Cherry GW, Harding KG, Ryan TJ, eds. Wound bed preparation. Proceedings of a symposium sponsored by the European Tissue Repair Society at St Anne's College and Green College, University of Oxford 2000. The Royal Society of Medicine Press, London

Thomas S, Fear M, Humphreys J *et al* (1996) The effect of dressings on the production of exudate from venous leg ulcers. *Wounds* **8**(5): 145–50

Thomas S (1997) Assessment and management of wound exudate. *J Wound Care* **6**(7): 327–30

Thomas D (2001) Matrix metalloproteinases, tissue inhibitors of metalloproteinases and wound bed status. In: Cherry GW, Harding KG, Ryan TJ, eds. Wound bed preparation. Proceedings of a symposium sponsored by the European Tissue Repair Society at St Anne's College and Green College, University of Oxford 2000. The Royal Society of Medicine Press, London

Trengove NJ, Langton SR, Stacey MC (1996) Biochemical analysis of wound fluid from non-healing and healing chronic leg ulcers. *Wound Repair Regen* **4**: 234–39

Vickery C (1997) Exudate: what is it and what is its function? In: Cherry GW, Harding K, eds. Management of Wound Exudate: Abstracts from the first combined meeting of the European Tissue Repair Society and the European Wound Management Association at Green College, University of Oxford. ETRS Bulletin)

Villavicencio RT (1998) The history of blue pus. *J Am Coll Surg* **187**(2): 212–6

White RJ (2001) Managing exudate. *Nurs Times* **97**: 9; XI–XIII

White RJ, Hothersall JS (2002) *The role of bacteria in promoting wound exudate: a hypothesis*. Presentation, Wounds-UK November 2002, Harrogate

Winter GD (1962) Formation of the scab and rate of epithelialisation of superficial wounds in the skin of the young domestic pig. *Nature* **193**: 293–4

Wysocki AB, Staiano-Coico L, Grinell F (1993) Wound fluid from chronic leg ulcers contains elevated levels of metalloproteinases MMP-2 and MMP-9. *J Investigative Dermat* **101**: 64–8

4

Skin grafts

Pauline Beldon

Part 1: Theory, procedure and management of graft sites in the community

The skin may not have the same the dramatic appeal as many of the other organs, such as the heart, however it plays a vital part in identifying each of us as a unique individual. When this protective outer barrier is damaged the consequences may be far reaching in both psychological and physical terms. Not all wounds require skin grafting — small, superficial wounds will heal by secondary intention and dressings. However, use of skin grafting to restore skin integrity for large surface wounds such as burns, reduces the risk of infection and enables the individual to resume normal daily activities more rapidly. The first part of this chapter explores the process of skin grafting and subsequent care of skin graft wound sites.

The skin is an organ with multiple functions. It is a highly resilient organ which in most cases can repair damage to itself with minimal intervention. However, where wounds are extensive, unsuitable for closure by suturing, or likely to cause physical or psychological problems through scarring, skin grafting may be considered to cover the wound, speed healing and minimize scarring.

In order to understand the use of different skin grafts for wound cover it is important to understand the anatomy of the skin in detail.

Functions of the skin

The skin is an outer covering for the internal structures of the body, and performs a number of functions (Mairis, 1992):

- the outer layer of epidermis is composed of keratin, which resists the action of all but the strongest acids and alkalis
- the skin maintains a stable environment preventing loss of water, electrolytes and proteins
- it absorbs ultraviolet radiation, stimulating production of vitamin D
- it aids temperature regulation by perspiration to cool the body and shivering to generate heat
- it excretes waste organic compounds and ions, water and heat in sweat
- its sensory function conveys information from the skin surface to the brain.
- the skin contains sensors for touch and pain, heat and cold.

Skin thickness varies during an individual's lifetime. The epidermis is at its thinnest at birth and in old age and at its thickest during puberty. The underlying dermis reaches maximum density during the individual's fourth decade, then gradually recedes (Ablove and Howell, 1997).

Structure of the skin

The skin is a complex structure divided into distinct layers: the epidermis, dermis, and subcutaneous layer. These are further subdivided into regions of cells which have particular roles in wound healing (*Figure 4.1*).

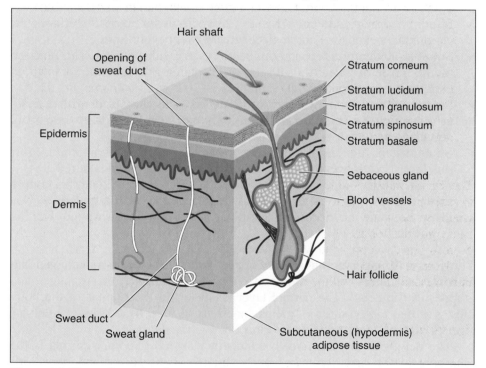

Figure 4.1: Three-dimensional cross section of the skin showing major structures and layers

The epidermis contains four major cell types:

✽ Keratinocytes, which produce the protein keratin in order to provide waterproofing of the skin and underlying tissue. These cells form the first line of defence against infection. At the base of the epidermis a germinative layer is constantly dividing, and new cells move upwards continually to replace the keratinocytes which are shed from the surface.

✽ Langerhans cells originate in the bone marrow and infiltrate the epidermis to assist with immunity. They are phagocytic, interact with the white blood cells, helper T-cells, in immune responses and secrete various substances which play a role in the wound healing process.

⌘ Melanocytes, contained in the deepest layer of the epidermis, produce the pigment melanin, which protects deeper tissues from the harmful effects of ultraviolet radiation.

⌘ Merkel cells are located in the stratum basale, where they are attached to keratinocytes. The cells are in close contact with the flattened ends of sensory neurones known as tactile discs, and are thought to relay the sensation of touch (Ablove and Howell, 1997).

The number of cell layers within the epidermis is dependant on the area of the body. Those areas which are in constant contact with friction, such as the palms and soles of feet, are covered by five cell layers:

⌘ Stratum corneum: twenty-five to thirty rows of dead keratinocytes, continually being shed and replaced every twenty-four hours.

⌘ Stratum lucidum: only found on the palms and soles of feet. The function of this layer of clear, flat, dead cells containing a substance known as eleidin, is to cushion impact.

⌘ Stratum granulosum: a layer of flattened cells involved with keratin formation, their nuclei are at various stages of degeneration as they break down and no longer perform a metabolic function.

⌘ Stratum spinosum: eight to ten rows of cells where keratin is produced. If this layer is permanently damaged scar tissue becomes discoloured.

⌘ Stratum basale: single layer of cuboidal to columnar cells. As they multiply they push upwards to become part of the upper layers of the epidermis. This layer is vital for fibroblast germination, essential in wound healing (Wysocki, 1995).

The dermis is mainly composed of connective tissue, containing collagen and elastin fibres. Cells within the dermis include fibroblasts, macrophages and adipocytes (fat cells). The dermal layer is thicker in those areas of the body most exposed to pressure, ie. palms and soles of feet. Blood vessels, nerves, sweat glands and hair follicles are embedded in the dermis.

The dermis is divided into two indistinct layers. Papillary dermis is the uppermost layer and comprises approximately one-fifth of the dermis. It consists of areolar connective tissue containing randomly organized, fine elastin, collagen and reticulin fibres. The surface area is greatly increased by the number of dermal papillae, finger-like projections with loops of capillaries. These infiltrate the epidermis and under the palms and soles of feet cause ridges in the overlying epidermis, ie. fingerprints. They also contain nerve endings for heat and cold detection.

The reticular dermis is the deeper layer, consisting mainly of dense irregular connective tissue containing bundles of collagen and elastin fibres. It is this layer which provides the skin with its elasticity and strength. Spaces between the fibres contain hair follicles, nerves, sweat and sebaceous glands and adipose tissue. If this layer is left intact in a wound, epidermal cells in the hair follicles and sweat and sebaceous glands will migrate across the wound surface to initiate epithelialization.

The reticular layer is attached to underlying bone and muscle by the subcutaneous layer which is constructed of adipocytes. Through this layer run the cutaneous nerves, blood and lymph vessels. Many of the cells found in the subcutaneous layer are capable of recognizing foreign antigens which may have been introduced into the skin.

Skin grafting

Skin grafting has been performed for thousands of years. In India around 2500–3000 years ago, skin was used to refashion noses which had been mutilated as punishment for adultery (Davis, 1941).

Skin grafting today is indicated by:

- loss of a large percentage of the skin, eg. as a result of burn or soft tissue trauma
- excision of benign or malignant lesions in areas of the body contraindicating direct closure by suturing, eg. basal cell carcinoma of the nasolabial fold of the nose
- excision of congenital problems, eg. large hairy naevus.

A skin graft is a section of epidermis and dermis which has been completely separated from its blood supply and donor site attachment before being transplanted to another area of the body, the recipient site (Grabb and Smith, 1991).

Classification

Classification of skin grafts may be based on the host-donor relationship and/or the thickness of dermis involved.

There are three classes of host-donor relationship:

- An autograft (autogenous) is when the donor and the recipient are the same individual.
- An allograft (homograft) occurs when the donor and the recipient are the same species, but different individuals.
- A xenograft (heterograft) describes a case where the donor and the recipient are different species. An example would be the use of material derived from cattle or pigs for human grafting.

The thickness of a split-skin graft will depend on the wound site and area of the body. For example, excision of burns scarring to the face will require a thinner graft than a wound on a limb, which is more prone to 'wear and tear' (McGregor and McGregor, 1995).

A full-thickness skin graft consists of epidermis and the full thickness of the dermis. The resultant defect is directly closed to heal by primary intention, since there remains no reticular dermis to initiate regeneration of epithelium. Donor sites are therefore chosen where a small area of skin may be directly excised and the resultant defect sutured, resulting in minimal scarring. Donor sites for full-thickness grafts include the post- and pre-auricular area; the supraclavicular area; the upper eyelid; the scalp; the antecubital and inguinal areas; and the areola (Nanchahal, 1999).

A split or partial-thickness skin graft involves excision of the epidermis and part of the dermis. Partial thickness grafts are further subdivided into:

- thin split-skin graft (0.008–0.012mm)
- intermediate split-skin graft (0.012–0.018mm)
- thick split-skin graft (0.018–0.030mm).

Because split-skin grafts leave 'islands' of reticular dermis at the donor site to permit regeneration of the skin (*Figure 4.2*), the surgeon can take larger areas of skin for the wound site. Donor sites for split skin grafts include: thigh and buttock; back; upper arm; forearm; and abdominal wall (Coull, 1991).

A skin graft is harvested from an area of the body that supplies a close match in skin texture, hair bearing, pigment and thickness to the recipient wound area. This is vital to produce both the best possible aesthetic result for the patient and appropriate thickness of graft to maintain skin integrity.

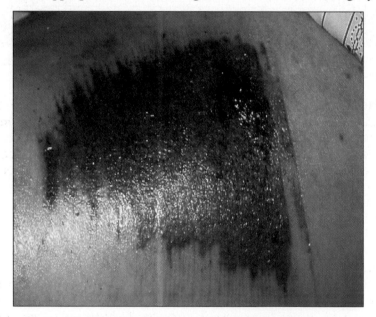

Figure 4.2: Almost-healed donor site on anterior thigh

Harvesting a skin graft

Skin grafts may be harvested using general or local anaesthesia. The skin is usually harvested using a dermatome, which permits a uniform excision and a quick procedure. (Freehand split-skin excisions are possible, but require great skill to achieve the correct thickness [*Figure 4.3*]). The dermatome holds a blade at a pre-set angle, which ensures the correct depth of skin is harvested. The skin is held at a constant, even tension ahead of the dermatome to aid an even excision.

Because they are taken from small areas, full thickness skin grafts, on the other hand, are usually harvested free hand using a scalpel.

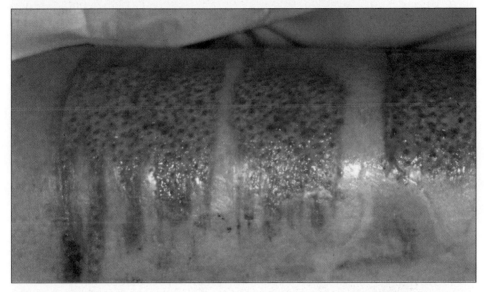

Figure 4.3: This donor site has been harvested freehand with a humby knife, hence the asymmetrical appearance

A degree of contracture occurs on harvesting a graft due to the elastic fibres in the dermis. Therefore, grafts with the thickest dermal layer contract most. If a thick dermal graft is applied over an unyielding area of the body, eg. scalp, little contracture is likely to occur. However, over an area which moves constantly due to underlying musculature, graft contracture may develop leading to unsightly scarring and/or reduced function of that area of the body.

Meshed skin grafts

A skin graft may be passed through a meshing device to insert multiple fenestrations into a graft. By permitting expansion of the graft tissue, meshing allows a graft to cover a larger surface area (*Figures 4.4, 5*). This, in turn, avoids the need for a large donor area, which would increase the insult to the skin integrity. In addition, if the wound is expected to bleed following surgery or produce copious amounts of serous fluid, a meshed graft allows this fluid to pass into the dressing freely and prevents the development of haematoma or seroma. The fenestrations rapidly re-epithelialize by secondary intention to provide complete skin cover. Meshed skin graft is, however, not suitable to cover all areas of the body as it retains the meshed appearance on healing; therefore, its use is avoided on the face, neck and hands (McGregor and McGregor, 1995).

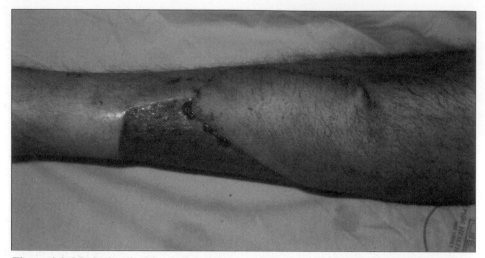

Figure 4.4: Meshed split skin graft applied to a defect resulting from the elevation of a right anterior fasciocutaneous flap. The graft is applied to the site from where the flap has been lifted

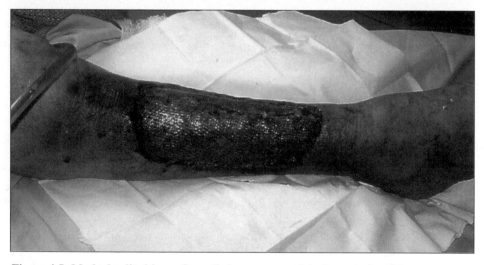

Figure 4.5: Meshed split skin graft applied over a wound to the anterior tibia

Attachment of the graft to recipient site

In order for the graft to adhere to the wound bed it must be held in close proximity and immobilized. This may be achieved by suturing the graft in place, both at the edges of the graft and centrally. Staples, clips and skin glue have also been used as rapid means of securing a graft in position. A firm dressing then holds the graft to ensure shearing (movement of the graft against the wound bed) does not occur.

A tie-over pack may be used to secure small grafts, especially to the head or neck area, or grafts placed into deep defects. Sutures are placed around the edge of the graft and the ends tied together over a pack of foam or sterile wool to ensure even pressure applied by the pack (Converse *et al*, 1975).

Factors affecting adherence of skin grafts

Successful adhesion depends on adequate arterial supply and venous drainage being established. Therefore the recipient wound bed should consist of only clean, viable tissue. The presence of any necrotic or sloughy tissue will necessitate surgical debridement in order to produce a good enough wound bed. Longstanding wounds may have chronic granulation present, which may be heavily colonized and have a mucoid surface, both of which may prevent graft adherence (Swaim, 1990).

Skin grafts will not adhere to bone, cartilage, tendon or nerve, which are deprived of their connective tissue covering. However, a skin graft will adhere well to bone covered with periosteum and cartilage with perichondrium (Nanchahal, 1999).

The presence of infection inhibits adherence because enzymes produced by bacteria, such as fibrinolysin, interfere with the normal fibrin attachment of the graft (Francis, 1998). The presence of haematoma or seroma acts as a barrier to adherence, therefore achieving haemostasis is essential at surgery. Pressure bandaging to limbs reduces the likelihood of this complication, as does elevation (McGregor and McGregor, 1995).

Physiology of skin graft adherence

Three phases have been described in skin graft adherence: serum imbibition, inosculation and revascularization (Swaim, 1990).

A fibrin network formed from the haemoserous fluid oozing from the wound bed adheres the graft to the wound bed very soon following application. As this contracts it pulls the graft into close contact with the wound bed. The fibrin network is then infiltrated by fibroblasts, leucocytes and phagocytes and is converted into a fibrous tissue attachment between the skin graft and wound bed. There follows a progressive gain in adherent strength between skin graft and wound bed. This continues until the fibrin network has been completely converted to fibrous tissue by approximately the tenth post-operative day (Swaim, 1990).

Serum imbibition

Serous fluid containing erythrocytes (red blood cells) and poly-morphonucleocytes accumulates between the skin graft and the wound bed. This results from plasma leakage from the venules in the wound bed. After the graft is applied the vessels in the graft dilate and capillary action draws serous fluid into them. Nutrition is therefore provided for the graft tissues and maintenance of dilated vessels is ensured until revascularization is achieved.

The graft has a white appearance at this time, as there are few erythrocytes present. Thinner grafts are more successful since the amount of nutrients able to reach the graft by serum imbibition is inversely proportional to the thickness of the graft (Swaim, 1990).

Inosculation

Inosculation occurs when vessels in the skin graft anastomose (join end-to-end) with vessels in the recipient wound bed of approximately the same diameter. This occurs twenty-four to seventy-two hours after application of the graft (Swaim, 1990). The fibrin network acts as a supportive framework along which endothelial buds from vessels in the recipient bed grow to meet the graft vessels. Blood flow through the anastomoses into the graft vessels occurs on day three to four and is sluggish until day five to six (Converse *et al*, 1975). The graft gradually takes on colour and becomes red/purple (thin-medium split skin graft) or pink/red (thick split skin and full thickness grafts (Converse *et al*, 1975).

Revascularization

Revascularization results from endothelial buds, which arise from arterioles, venules and capillaries in both the wound bed and the skin graft. From each bud, a cord of endothelial cells grows into the dermis of the graft and anastomoses with graft vessel or another endothelial cord. Maturation of vessels begins approximately forty-eight hours following the appearance of new capillaries, and maturation and differentiation continues until a system of arterioles, venules and capillaries is formed (Pope, 1988). Lymph vessels also develop; the lymph system is usually established by day four to five (Swaim, 1990).

As the graft continues to mature in its new site, it is partially innervated by the sensory nerves of the wound bed. Split-skin grafts are innervated more quickly than full-thickness skin grafts but not as completely. This is thought to be due to the thickness of the skin graft (Branham and Thomas, 1990). Any surgical procedure is likely to result in altered sensation, including skin grafting (McGregor and McGregor, 1995).

Scar contracture occurs gradually over the next six to twelve months. The thicker the graft, the less contracture occurs (Branham and Thomas, 1990).

First inspection of skin graft

Following surgery, the time period which elapses until first inspection of the skin graft varies depending on; the site of the graft, its thickness, means of immobilization, aetiology of the defect site, age of the patient, existence of underlying medical condition which could delay healing, etc. In other words, there is no fixed time. However an estimation can be made for each individual patient, taking into consideration all of the above factors. Generally, the first postoperative dressing change is performed two to five days after surgery (Young and Fowler, 1998).

With the development of plastic surgery liaison/outreach nurses, the first dressing change is being performed more commonly in the community setting (Beldon, 1992). This provides community nurses with the opportunity to care for skin grafts in the acute phase of healing.

A patient may not be experiencing pain at the graft site, but they may feel very anxious. Experience suggests a great emphasis is always placed on the first inspection of a graft and whether or not it has succeeded. Patients feel the sense of occasion, so it is important to outline — as realistically as possible — how the graft site might appear, in order to avoid the patient feeling great disappointment. The graft is not going to have the same appearance as the surrounding skin; it is likely to appear red/mauve in colour due to inosculation and revascularization. If a large amount of devitalised tissue or a lesion has been removed, there may be a significant depression to the normal outline, which may dismay the patient. If the presence of infection is suspected, the patient should be warned that none of the skin graft may have survived.

On first inspecting a skin graft site it is important to remove the overlying dressings with care. Occasionally, dressings are firmly adhered to the graft by dried blood or exudate and may need to be soaked away. Clumsy removal of the dressing can traumatize the new vascularity of the graft. If it is suspected that a dressing has closely adhered to a wound bed then advice should be sought from a plastic surgery department or tissue viability nurse.

Whether the graft has successfully adhered or not will be determined by:

⌘ Colour: A thin–medium split-skin graft should be red/mauve as a result of inosculation and revascularization. A thick split-skin graft or a full thickness graft may be pink/red in colour due to the density of the graft.
⌘ Immobility: On placing a gloved finger onto the graft it should not be mobile but firmly adhered to the underlying wound bed.

The percentage of skin graft which has adhered successfully to the wound bed is estimated as an indicator of the procedure's success. A completely covered wound with immobile, vascularized graft is deemed to have 100% coverage.

Whether or not the skin graft has adhered to the wound bed, all sutures, staples or glue should be removed. Their purpose has been served. There is nothing to be gained from leaving dissolvable sutures *in situ*, they may act as an irritant and detract from the aesthetic result (McGregor and McGregor, 1995).

The surgeon will have overlapped the wound edges with skin graft, in order to ensure the wound bed will still be covered should the graft contract. These edges will have desiccated and should be trimmed away. Any small seroma that may be present, should be perforated and expressed (Converse *et al*, 1975).

Subsequent dressings for skin grafts depend on the percentage of graft cover, the amount of exudate produced, the presence of infection, practicality and site of the body. A graft that has completely adhered to a wound bed should be regarded as a healed wound since skin integrity has been restored. As such, it no longer requires dressings. For example, a full-thickness skin graft to the head/neck will be left exposed and the patient advised to wash and pat dry the area. Gentle massage with a non-perfumed emollient is advised to aid the graft site to become supple and move with the facial muscles (Young and Fowler, 1998).

Partial wound healing

A successful graft adherence to a whole wound might be expected in a young, healthy individual with no underlying medical problems. However, an older patient with ageing skin physiology may be less fortunate, and partial wound healing is a common result.

Continued wound management is then dictated by a number of factors:

- the cause of partial success, eg. the presence of heavy colonization or infection, haematoma, partial shearing of graft
- the percentage of skin graft cover to the wound
- the amount of exudate produced
- wound site
- practicality.

Of the factors listed above, the single most important is exudate. This usually dictates both the frequency of dressing change and the absorbency of the dressings.

Non-adherent dressings are simple and practical to use, and are easily removed at dressing changes. Provided only a small amount of exudate is produced by the graft site, renewal of dressings may then occur infrequently, allowing the wound to continue re-epithelialization undisturbed.

Hydrocolloid dressings aid rapid re-epithelialization by providing a moist, occlusive environment. However, hypergranulation has been known to occur under hydrocolloids (Young, 1995), so these should be used with caution. Should any of the graft have necrosed, usually due to either infection or excessive pressure, then a hydrocolloid dressing is useful in debriding this area by autolysis without traumatizing the remaining graft (Thomas and Leigh, 1998).

If moderate-large amounts of exudate are produced then an alginate dressing or hydrofibre dressing may be appropriate. These can absorb large quantities of exudate without causing maceration of the graft (Thomas and Loveless, 1992). If the graft site is to a lower leg and is heavily exuding then the limb should be examined for varicose veins and a comprehensive leg ulcer assessment performed, including Doppler ultrasound (Fronek, 1989), as excessive exudate may result from oedema caused by venous disease. Such wounds may benefit from compression therapy.

Any partially healed skin graft site is at risk from infection since it remains an open wound. Infection is a common cause if only a small percentage of the graft has adhered to the wound bed. In this instance, the practitioner should treat the wound as an infected wound – the presence of some adhered skin graft does not alter treatment. Consequently, antimicrobial wound management products may be used together with systemic antibiotics.

Common complications in managing skin grafts, donor sites and wounds

Problem	Nursing action	Rationale
Suspected infection Patient has malaise and pyrexia Wound is inflamed, malodorous Producing purulent exudate, increasing in size and exhibiting general deterioration	Inform patient and surgeon of suspicion Wound swab for culture and sensitivity to antibiotics Assess wound, are symptoms reminiscent of common infection Apply appropriate wound product to treat symptoms topically or relieve discomfort. Redress daily, documenting accurately status of patient and wound	Communication Identification of bacteria, ensure appropriate antibiotic therapy Baseline information. Possible to identify common infections Dual action of treatment with systemic antibiotics Monitor progress
Wound is heavily exudating (infection not suspected)	Assess wound. Does patient have underlying systemic problem? Is surrounding skin in tact? Apply moisture repellent to skin, eg. Cavilon™ barrier cream or soft paraffin Identify type of exudate, ie. serous fluid Apply appropriate wound management product to absorb exudate while maintaining some moisture at wound site For example, hydrofibre, foam or alginate dressing Change dressings when strikethrough observed at outer dressing Document efficacy of dressing and wound progress	Baseline information, ie. if leg wound, does patient have venous insufficiency Determine effect of exudate on skin ? danger of maceration Hydro-absorptive products Prevent maceration of surrounding skin Monitor progress
On first inspection the graft/donor site is partially healed. Low or nil exudate	Assess wound, estimate percentage without skin cover Apply appropriate wound management product to provide moist environment For example, hydrocolloid as primary dressing or hydrogel as primary dressing with secondary dressing Change dressing infrequently	Baseline information To encourage proliferation of epithelium Water-donating products Choice may be decided by wound site
Non-healing donor site in excess of three weeks	Reassess wound to determine cause Wound swab for culture and sensitivity Apply wound management product appropriate for amount of exudate produced	? Inappropriate dressing applied ? Friction forces applied at wound bed possibility of critical colonisation/infection To absorb exudate while maintaining moist environment necessary for re-epithilialization
Hypergranulation tissue present in graft or donor site	Caused by insufficient speed of re-epithelialization Choice of products: pressure via foam dressing hydrocortisone 1% ointment or Terra-Cortril™ ointment	Mechanical suppression of hypergranulation Reduce fibroblast activity

Conclusion

Skin is the normal covering of the body; accordingly the aim of a surgeon employing skin grafting techniques is to restore skin cover when an insult to its integrity occurs. Wounds without the benefit of skin cover are at risk from infection, reduce the function of that area and prevent normal living. The application of a skin graft may not always be completely successful, but will invariably shorten healing time for the patient (Kirsner *et al*, 1993), thereby reducing the possibility of infection and returning the patient to normal lifestyle more quickly.

Skin grafts are now routinely applied to wound beds as an outpatient procedure, especially following excision of suspected lesions. Consequently more nurses in community and practice settings are likely to encounter these specialist wounds with their unusual dressing – skin. How these wounds are subsequently managed is reliant on the practitioner's recognition of skin grafts and knowledge of their management, together with good wound management practice based on robust evidence.

The next part of this chapter will discuss care of the second wound site in any grafting procedure: the donor site.

Key points

⌘ Good knowledge of the anatomy of the skin is vital in order to understand the difference in different skin grafts and the role that various cells play in wound healing.

⌘ Skin grafting is appropriate for large superficial and deep wounds which may otherwise have prolonged healing times.

⌘ Care of skin grafts is increasingly taking place in the community, so a knowledge of the processes of and hindrances to graft adhesion and integrity is important.

References

Ablove RH, Howell RM (1997) The physiology and technique of skin grafting. *Hand Clin* **13**(2): 163–73

Beldon P (1992) Plastic surgery liaison nursing. *Community Outlook* **July:** 21–3

Branham GH, Thomas JR (1990) Skin grafts: facial plastic surgery. *Otolaryngol Clin North Am* **23**(5): 889–97

Converse JM, Smahel J, Ballantyne DL Jr, Harper AD (1975) Inosculation of vessels of skin graft and host bed: a fortuitous encounter. *Br J Plast Surg* **28**(4): 274-82

Coull A (1991) Making sense of split skin graft donor sites. *Nurs Times* **87**(40): 52–4

Davis JS (1910) Skin transplantation. *John Hopkins Hosp Rep* **15:** 307

Davis JS (1941) The story of plastic surgery. *Ann Surg* **113:** 641

Francis A (1998) Nursing management of skin graft sites. *Nurs Stand* **12**(33): 41–4

Fronek A (1989) *Non-invasive Diagnostics in Vascular Disease*. McGraw-Hill, New York

Grabb WC, Smith JW (1991) *Plastic Surgery*. 3rd edn. Little Brown, Boston

Kirsner RS, Falanga V, Eaglstein WH (1993) The biology of skin grafts. Skin grafts as pharmacologic agents. *Arch Dermatology* **129**(4): 481–3

McGregor A, McGregor I (1995) *Fundamental Techniques of Plastic Surgery*. Churchill Livingstone, Edinburgh

Mairis E (1992) Four senses for a full skin assessment; observation and assessment of the skin. *Prof Nurse* **7**(6): 376–80

Nanchahal J (1999) Skin loss: grafts and flaps. *Surgery* **17**(4): 76–80

Pope ER (1988) Skin grafting in small animal surgery. Part 1: The normal healing process. *Compendium of Continuing Education* **10**: 1068

Swaim SF (1990) Skin grafts. *Vet Clin North Am Small Anim Pract* **20**(1): 147–75

Thomas S, Leigh IM (1998) Wound dressings. In: Leaper DJ, Harding KG, eds. *Wounds: Biology and Management*. Oxford University Press, Oxford: 1734

Thomas A, Loveless PJ (1992) Observations of the fluid handling properties of alginate dressings. *Pharmaceutical J* **247**: 850–1

Young T (1995) Common problems in overgranulation. *Practice Nurse* **6**(11): 14–16

Young T, Fowler A (1998) Nursing management of skin grafts and donor sites. *Br J Nurs* **7**(6): 324–330

Weber RS, Hankins P, Limitone E, Callender D (1995) Split skin graft donor site management. *Arch Otolaryngol Head Neck Surgery* **121**: 1145–9

Wysocki A (1995) A review of the skin and its appendages. *Adv Wound Care* **8**(2) Part I: 53–64

Part 2: Management of donor site wounds in the community

Skin grafting is a surgical procedure used to quickly restore skin integrity in large wounds or those wounds which cannot be directly closed by suturing. The procedure of skin grafting necessitates the creation of a second wound; the donor site. Although often viewed as secondary importance by surgeons once skin has been harvested from the area, it is the donor site which frequently causes complications such as pain/discomfort and slow healing (Wilkinson, 1997). Because skin graft sites and donor sites are viewed as part of a specialist practice, their wound management is regarded as being 'something different'. However, the donor site is a partial-dermal thickness wound and should be seen as such, rather than a 'special' wound. This may help to lessen the anxiety felt by both patient and nurse in dealing with donor site wounds.

Patients discharged from plastic surgery, and other specialist units where skin grafting is employed, may have two wounds referred to the care of the community nurse, the graft site and the donor site. Often, the patient's attention is focused not on the original wound, the recipient of the skin graft, but on the donor site from which the skin graft was taken. This is normally because the donor site causes more discomfort and produces high levels of exudate initially, often requiring several dressings, which the patient may recall with pain unless their analgesic needs have been addressed. Once home, the patient requires a practical dressing, which allows freedom of movement, reduced risk of staining clothing, can be removed infrequently without discomfort and will aid healing.

Because skin graft sites and donor sites are viewed as part of a specialist practice, their wound management is regarded as being 'something different'. However, the donor site is a partial-dermal thickness wound and should be seen as such, rather than a 'special' wound.

Donor sites

A donor site is an area of the body from which skin has been harvested to provide a split-skin graft. The graft comprises the epidermis and a partial-thickness of the reticular dermis, leaving behind a portion of the reticular dermis, which contains partial hair follicles and sebaceous glands, to enable spontaneous re-epithelialization of the donor site area to occur. The patient then has a superficial wound, exposing the dermis and nerve endings (*Figure 4.6*).

The main considerations for choice of donor site are:

- the skin tone/colour and texture — usually the closer the donor site is to the primary wound the closer the skin 'match'
- how large a skin graft is needed
- how visible the resultant scar will be on that area of the body.

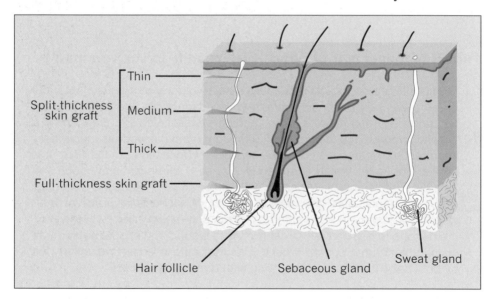

Figure 4.6: Relative thicknesses of split-skin and full-thickness skin grafts

The patient will have been made aware before the operation of the need to inflict another wound to produce the skin graft; also that a donor site may be more painful, initially, than the original wound because of exposure of sensory nerve endings and that regular analgesia will be prescribed. It has been frequently reported that donor sites cause patients more pain and discomfort than the recipient wound site (Weber *et al*, 1995). It is this factor and the amount of exudate produced which can render donor site healing problematic. The patient should be consulted regarding the site of the donor site. A patient may prefer to have a wound on their buttock, rather than the anterior thigh, because the resultant pale square/rectangular scar will be less visible (*Figure 4.7*). Common areas for split skin donor sites include the thigh (most common), buttock, back, upper arm and abdominal wall.

The procedure of skin graft harvest

During surgery, an emollient such as liquid paraffin may be applied to the skin to minimize damage to the skin at the edges of the donor site, owing to friction from the dermatome or knife used to harvest the graft (Swaim, 1990). The skin graft is then removed from the patient and stored ready for application to the original wound. The surgeon may then sprinkle the wound with a haemostatic agent, eg. a topical adrenaline or local anaesthetic like lignocaine, to reduce immediate postoperative bleeding and effect some pain relief. A dressing is then applied and the donor site sealed.

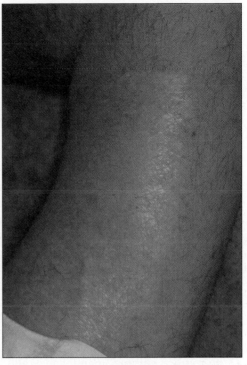

Healing

Figure 4.7: A healed donor site, which is hairless and a lighter colour than surrounding skin

Healing of the split-skin donor site occurs through re-epithelialization — epithelial cells migrate from the adnexal processes of the skin, the sebaceous and sweat glands and hair follicles. They then migrate and proliferate across the wound to restore skin integrity. How long this process takes varies; a young patient may heal in seven to ten days, however healing may take up to three weeks in an older patient (Fatah and Ward, 1984). Healing is dependant on factors such as the depth of the donor site, how much of the reticular dermis remains, the surface area of the wound, nutritional status and prevention of infection (Young and Fowler, 1998).

If an older patient has a large donor site wound, a small piece of the skin graft can be widely fenestrated (meshed), producing an effect much like fishnet stockings (*Figure 4.8*). This is replaced onto the donor site as an ideal autologous, biological dressing, a restorative dressing, enabling keratinocytes to spread out from the graft across the wound site and speed healing via re-epithelialization.

In the first three to four days after surgery, the wound may produce copious serous exudate, dependant on the surface area, which then dramatically falls to a minimum as re-epithelialization progresses. Initially, therefore, the choice of dressing is based on the absorbent qualities of the dressing. Traditionally, paraffin gauze has been used as a primary dressing for donor areas, with an absorbent secondary dressing such as gauze or wool, then pressure applied via a crepe bandage to aid haemostasis (Brotherston and Lawrence, 1993). However, paraffin gauze adheres closely to the wound and on drying out becomes difficult to remove, causing discomfort and trauma to the wound bed. Furthermore, if left for seven to ten days there is a tendency for epithelium to become incorporated into the dressing (*Figure 4.9*) (Fowler and Dempsey, 1998; Porter, 1991). While many plastic surgery units have now moved away from using paraffin gauze dressings, other specialities using skin grafting have not (Edwards *et al*, 1998).

In the last twenty years there has been a move towards wound management products which facilitate the body's own efforts in healing. This would appear to contraindicate the continued use of paraffin gauze dressings, certainly for donor site management if not in other areas of wound management.

The growing awareness of the discomfort suffered by patients on removal of dressings indicates the need for more careful, informed choice of wound management products to prevent traumatizing both patient and the wound bed on removal (European Wound Management Association, 2002).

The main principles of a wound management product, in this context, are:

- to protect the area from dehydration once exudate production falls
- to prevent further mechanical trauma
- to reduce pain
- to minimize leakage of exudate (Weber *et al*, 1995)
- to promote rapid, infection-free healing
- to be practical to apply and remove
- to require minimal maintenance and be inexpensive.

It may be possible that the first choice of donor site dressing will be appropriate until the wound is healed. However, when the exudate levels fall, approximately three to four days after surgery, the original choice of dressing should be reviewed and possibly changed to one which will maintain a moist occlusive environment until full skin integrity has been achieved.

Appropriate dressings

Hydrocolloid dressings

Hydrocolloids will absorb low-to-moderate levels of exudate, provided a large enough sheet is used. Hydrocolloids have been found useful when the exudate levels fall to minimum, as the dressing will maintain the moist environment necessary for re-epithelialization (Doherty *et al*, 1986). Hydrocolloid dressings require no secondary dressing and allow patients to shower. In the initial stages, the amount of exudate is probably too great for absorption by a hydrocolloid – such a dressing would necessitate frequent changes and become impractical and costly (Bettinger *et al*, 1995).

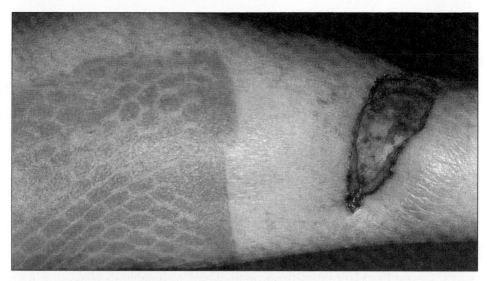

Figure 4.8: Widely-meshed skin graft applied to donor site

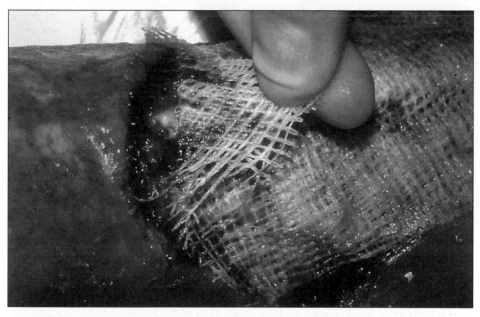

Figure 4.9: Example of new tissue growing into gauze dressing, resulting in pain and trauma on removal

Alginate dressings

An alginate dressing will act as a haemostat and absorb exudate initially, however if re-applied when exudate levels fall, it may not maintain sufficient moisture at the wound surface, leading to drying and delayed healing (Brady *et al*, 1980).

Hydrofibre

Hydrofibre acts as a haemostat. It absorbs excess moisture and binds water molecules permanently onto the hydrocolloid molecule, transforming the dressing into a gel-like sheet which maintains a moist wound environment.

Foam

Foam dressings draw excess moisture away from the wound by capillary action. Foams have a low adherence to the wound bed. In addition, they retain large volumes of exudate and provide patient comfort, suggesting they have a role to play in donor site management (Wilkinson, 1997).

Semi-permeable films

Semi-permeable films are commonly used as a secondary dressing. They allow water vapour to escape from the wound. They are unable to cope with high levels of exudate so are inappropriate initially, but as exudate levels fall may be comfortable for the patient (James and Watson, 1975).

Non-adherent silicone and polyamide net

These dressings allow excess exudate to pass through into secondary dressing, which is then changed as needed, leaving the primary dressing *in situ* until healed. Platt *et al* (1996) noted that non-adherent silicone dressings were significantly easier to remove than alginate dressings and do not shed fibres into the wound bed.

Example one

An elderly patient has a donor site on the anterior thigh, approximately 10cm by 15cm. In theatre, the surgeon has applied an alginate dressing after sprinkling the wound with local anaesthetic. This has then been covered with gauze roll and a firm crepe bandage to apply pressure. The alginate will be saturated with haemoserous exudate in a short time, but the dressing should be left *in situ*, since removing the dressing and relieving the pressure may cause more discomfort to the patient and allow greater exudate production than would otherwise occur.

After twenty-four to forty-eight hours, the pressure may be released, the primary alginate dressing changed and a semi-permeable film dressing applied. This will allow the patient to mobilize without fear of the dressing slipping and allows nursing staff to observe when the alginate is fully saturated with exudate.

An alginate might possibly remain the dressing of choice until full healing has occurred. However, if on dressing change the wound appears partially re-epithelialized and incapable of producing exudate, it would perhaps be appropriate to apply a dressing such as a hydrocolloid which will maintain sufficient moisture at the wound surface to permit continued proliferation of the epithelium.

Care of the donor site

Fowler and Dempsey (1998) have described comprehensively the appropriate nursing management of donor sites:

⌘ Administer analgesia as prescribed regularly. Inform surgeon or GP if appears inadequate.
⌘ Aid pain management and haemostasis through elevation and/or immobilization of donor site area.
⌘ Observe and act on signs of excessive bleeding, infection, pain unrelieved by analgesia, pyrexia, malodorous wound site.
⌘ Reassure the patient regarding wound odour, which can be embarrassing. Explain this is related to stale blood or exudate trapped in the dressing. This may be improved by increasing the frequency of dressing change.
⌘ Remove the dressing before the agreed date only if it is grossly contaminated, review the initial primary dressing choice and change to anti-microbial agent if necessary.
⌘ Ensure choice of dressing is practical, does not impede mobility and remains *in situ*. Dressings which slip cause unnecessary friction and wound damage
⌘ Allow primary contact layer to separate spontaneously, never soak or pull.
⌘ Classify a donor site as healed only if the primary contact layer is removed without pain leaving a dry, re-epithelialized surface.
⌘ Ensure the patient has appropriate advice regarding aftercare.

Often when a community nurse takes over patient care, the donor site is partially healed and the exudate levels have considerably reduced. The patient may have become used to the initial dressing used in hospital and may not understand the reason for change. Communication is therefore a key skill at this time, to translate the information from the nurse's wound assessment into lay terms for the patient.

Example two

A thirty-six-year-old male has an extensive donor site of 20cm by 15cm over his anterior and lateral thigh. On discharge from hospital at six days after surgery the donor site is partially healed and re-epithelializing, producing low-to-moderate amounts of exudate. The patient complains of being unable to shower and the donor site is uncomfortable. A bordered foam dressing will act as both primary and secondary dressing and may be left *in situ* for up to several days. The wound contact layer is a heat-treated polyurethane surface, preventing adherence of new epithelium and providing a comfortable sealed environment for the patient.

The infected donor site

Signs of infection are the same as for most other wounds:

- pyrexia
- raised white cell count
- inflammation
- increased/altered pain/discomfort
- increased exudate
- altered odour
- wound bed bleeds easily
- pocketing at base of the wound
- bridging of epithelium
- wound breakdown (Cutting and Harding, 1994).

The patient is a reliable witness of their own condition. If they report a change in sensation/pain, increase in exudate and a malodour, then the nurse should check for pyrexia and raised white cell count and remove the dressing to examine the wound.

Should a donor site become infected (*Figure 4.10*) it should be treated as any other infected partial-thickness wound. A topical antimicrobial (eg. silver sulphadiazine) or a silver-impregnated dressing may be useful.

If any partial-dermal thickness wound becomes infected, there is always the risk of the wound becoming deeper. If it then becomes a full-dermal thickness wound it will be very slow to heal, as epithelium will only be able to travel from the edges of the wound. In this case, the patient may require another skin graft to be applied to the donor site.

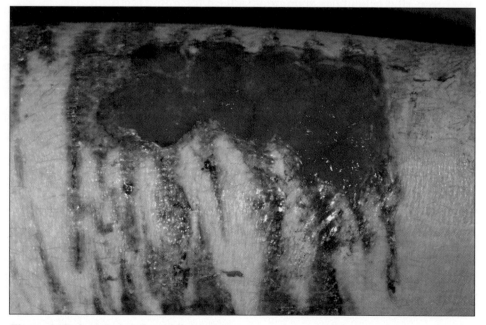

Figure 4.10: An infected donor site wound

Patient advice following healing of donor sites

Patients may be anxious regarding their own care of their donor site. It will have been a painful wound, and although it may heal rapidly it still causes concern.

Initially, the epithelium over the newly healed donor area may be dry and itchy. However, scratching must be avoided, as nails can traumatize the new epithelium. Keeping the area cool may help this. In extreme cases, antihistamines have helped (Francis, 1998). The patient should be advised to wash the area using a non-perfumed soap or an emollient and gentle pressure for the first few weeks. Application of a non-perfumed moisturiser will keep the area supple and reduce dryness. Commonly used preparations include E45® (Crookes Healthcare) and Diprobase® (Schering-Plough); however, both these products contain lanolin or lanolin derivatives which may lead to skin sensitivity. An alternative is 50% liquid paraffin/50% white soft paraffin, which is easily absorbed and excipient-free.

Patients should be advised to avoid sunbathing and to apply a total sun block for the first year after surgery to avoid burning (Fowler and Dempsey, 1998). Chlorinated swimming pools have also been known to cause irritation so should be avoided for the first few weeks after healing is complete.

Conclusion

Donor site wounds often cause patients and community nurses problems owing to discomfort and management of exudate from a flat superficial wound bed. However, the donor site wound should be treated as any other large partial-dermal thickness wound. Analgesia is vital, initially, then less so as the wound progresses towards healing. What patients desire is a comfortable dressing, which will allow them to shower, and be changed only infrequently to allow them to return to normal daily living. Community nurses have many wound management products available on prescription to help them achieve this aim.

Key points

⌘ Donor site wounds are partial-dermal thickness wounds left to heal by secondary intention.

⌘ Patients identify pain/discomfort and exudate as their main concerns for management.

⌘ No one wound management product is ideal to manage a donor site wound; choice is dictated by the assessment of the individual patient.

References

Bettinger D, Gore D, Humphries Y (1995) Evaluation of calcium alginate for skin graft donor sites. *J Burn Care Rehabil* **16**(1): 59–61

Brady SC, Snelling CF, Chow G (1980) Comparison of donor site dressings. *Ann Plast Surg* **5**(3): 238–43

Brotherston TM, Lawrence JC (1993) Dressings for donor sites. *J Wound Care* **2**(2): 84–8

Cutting KF, Harding KG (1994) Criteria for identifying wound infection. *J Wound Care* **3**(4): 198–201

Doherty C, Lynch G, Noble S (1986) Granuflex hydrocolloid as a donor site dressing. *Care of the Critically Ill* **2:** 193–4

Edwards H, Gaskill D, Nash R (1998) Treating skin tears in nursing home residents: a pilot study comparing four types of dressings. *Int J Nursing Practice* **4**(1): 25–32

European Wound Management Association (2002) *A Position Document: Pain at Wound Dressing Changes*. Medical Education Partnership Ltd, London

Fatah M, Ward CM (1984) The morbidity of split skin graft donor sites in the elderly: the case for mesh grafting the donor site. *Br J Plast Surg* **37**(2): 184–90

Fowler A, Dempsey A (1998) Split-thickness skin graft donor sites. *J Wound Care* **7**(8): 399–402

Francis A (1998) Nursing management of skin graft sites. *Nurs Stand* **12**(33): 41–4

James JH, Watson AC (1975) The use of Opsite, a vapour permeable dressing on skin graft donor sites. *Br J Plast Surg* **28**(2): 107–10

Platt AJ, Phipps A, Judkins K (1996) A comparative study of silicone net dressing and paraffin gauze dressing in skin grafted sites. *Burns* **22**(7): 543–5

Porter JM (1991) A comparative investigation of re-epithelialization of split-skin donor sites after application of hydrocolloid and alginate dressings. *Br J Plast Surg* **44**(5): 333–7

Swaim SF (1990) Skin grafts. *Vet Clin North Am* **20**(1): 147–75

Weber RS, Hankins P, Limitone E *et al* (1995) Split thickness skin graft donor site management. A randomized prospective trial comparing a hydrophilic polyurethane absorbent foam dressing with a petrolatum gauze dressing. *Arch Otolaryngol Head Neck Surg* **121**(10): 1145–9

Wilkinson B (1997) Hard graft. *Nurs Times* **93**(16): 63–9

Young T, Fowler A (1998) Nursing management of skin grafts and donor sites. *Br J Nurs* **7**(6): 324-6

5

Managing patients unable to tolerate therapeutic compression

Sue Bale, Keith G Harding

Managing patients with venous ulceration who are unable to tolerate therapeutic compression bandaging is a challenging clinical problem. This study followed a group of twenty-eight such patients who were treated with three layers of graduated Tubigrip as an alternative to therapeutic compression. It also investigated factors that influenced nurses in deciding to use this bandaging system. Patients were followed until their ulcers healed or for a maximum of twelve weeks. The decision to use three layers of graduated Tubigrip was based on nineteen patients' desire to wear their normal shoes (67.9%) and the convenience of access to the ulcer by eight patients (28.6%) (to permit frequent dressing changes for large or infected ulcers, and for the daily application of steroidal creams to peri-ulcer skin). Fourteen patients' ulcers had healed within the twelve-week study period. The remaining fourteen patients had a mean reduction in ulcer area of 4.6cm^2 (SD=7.4), and median of 2.3cm^2 (range 28.5).The authors found three layers of graduated Tubigrip useful for managing patients who cannot tolerate therapeutic forms of compression.

Providing care for patients with venous leg ulceration, who may take months to achieve healing, can be frustrating, time-consuming and expensive. In the community, district nurses, practice nurses and GPs usually care for this group of patients and are responsible for providing appropriate, effective treatment. For patients with venous leg ulceration, compression therapy is recommended as the best treatment option (Fletcher *et al*, 1997) and high compression has been shown to be better than low compression (Fletcher *et al*, 1997).

Some patients are referred to specialist leg ulcer clinics (Moffatt and Dickson, 1993) for advice and treatment for complex clinical problems. In the authors' experience, not all patients referred to a specialist leg ulcer clinic are able to tolerate the high levels of compression required to be therapeutic. This is often owing to a negative past experience with compression. This can create problems for nurses and doctors who are trying to provide effective treatment. Selim *et al* (2001) discussed the problem of delivering evidence-based care when a patient was unable to accept the recommended treatment. In this instance this was because of personal preference. They described how evidence-based practice had to be modified to deliver client-focused care that best met the emotional and physical needs of this patient.

Problems arise in making clinical decisions when patients' wishes are at odds with the recommendations for delivering evidence-based care, and that evidence is only one factor that influences decisions about patient care.

The process of making clinical decisions is complex and several authors have suggested factors that might influence clinicians (Haynes and Haines, 1998; Closs and Cheater, 1999). Haynes and Haines cite resource availability, the experience of the clinician, the risk of adverse outcomes and patient circumstances and preferences. Closs and Cheater focus on patient preference and argue that the degree to which a patient's preference will be accommodated is influenced by the practitioner's clinical experience, personal attitudes, values and beliefs, the potential risk of adverse reactions, and the professional opinions of colleagues' knowledge of the extent of the problem.

Taking account of individual patient circumstances and patient preference is recognized by Coulter (2000) as becoming increasingly important in encouraging patient concordance (in the past reported as patient compliance) with treatment. Government recommendations also emphasize the role of patients and support the principle of encouraging patients to participate in their own care (Department of Health [DoH], 1997). Douglas (2001) reported the results of a qualitative study that explored patients' experiences of leg ulceration and described the benefits of working in partnership with patients.

This chapter reports on the results of a study that followed a group of twenty-eight patients attending a specialist wound healing clinic who were unable to tolerate therapeutic compression bandaging, which is often owing to a negative past experience with compression. The study investigated the factors that influenced nurses in making decisions about these patients' treatment.

History and background

The Wound Healing Research Unit in Cardiff has provided a service for patients with leg ulceration in an outpatient clinic for the past twenty-two years, working closely with GPs and district and practice nurses. In line with other leg ulcer services (Morison and Moffatt, 1994; Falanga, 1997; Doughty *et al*, 2000), a full patient assessment is combined with offering patients a range of investigation and treatment options. Because of the tertiary nature of the referral, patients presenting to this specialist service with venous ulceration have frequently had prior experience of compression bandaging.

Some patients' experience of compression bandaging has not always been positive and has led to them refusing compression. Managing this difficult clinical situation is a challenge as patient concordance with compression is considered an essential element of successful treatment. In the authors' experience, these patients require a more pragmatic and flexible approach, where a gradual introduction to compression may be more successful in their management.

Using three layers of graduated Tubigrip

The authors have devised and had experience of using three layers of graduated Tubigrip in the Wound Healing Research Unit to introduce patients to compression. This system has also been used in treating patients who are non-concordant with compression bandaging in the longer term. Initially, patients are fitted with Tubigrip one size larger than they require to help them gain confidence and to prevent discomfort. Patients reported that the Tubigrip was comfortable when applied in three graduated layers and had the advantage of being easily removed (when discomfort occurred) and reapplied later. The authors have found that empowering this group of patients to be in control of their bandages can encourage them to persevere with treatment.

Having gained confidence, some patients progressed to standard compression systems (eg. four-layer bandaging or wool and Class III bandages), and others were fitted with tighter three-layer graduated Tubigrip. Empowering patients and encouraging them to become equal partners in their care is recommended by Coulter (2000) as one route towards ensuring that patients make the most effective use of health services.

All patients had their legs measured (at the widest point of the ankle and calf) to determine the correct size of Tubigrip needed to achieve high compression. The Tubigrip was applied in three layers (*Figure 5.1*):

⌘ Layer 1: from the metatarsal heads to the tibial tuberosity
⌘ Layer 2: from the metatarsal heads to mid-calf
⌘ Layer 3: from the metatarsal heads to the origin of the Achilles tendon.

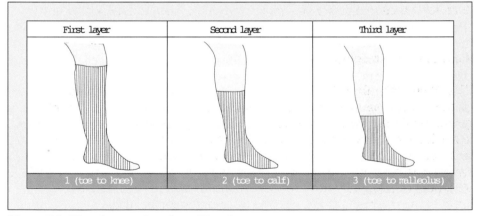

Figure 5.1: Three layers of graduated bandage

Objectives

The main objective of this study was to measure the effect of using this treatment on healing and reduction in ulcer area. It also explored the factors that influenced nurses to select three layers of graduated Tubigrip for patients who were unable to tolerate therapeutic levels of compression.

Methods

A prospective, non-comparative study of patients with venous leg ulceration presenting to a specialist leg ulcer clinic who were unable to tolerate therapeutic compression owing to negative past experience, were selected for treatment with three layers of graduated Tubigrip.

A purposive sampling technique was employed. Purposive sampling is recommended when researchers wish to study the effects of a new treatment on a specific group of patients (Bowling, 1997), in this case patients who are unable to tolerate therapeutic compression. The results cannot be generalizable to the wider population (in this case to all patients with leg ulceration). Patients were assessed at four time points: on entry to the study, then at weeks four, eight and twelve. Patients were followed for twelve weeks or until their wounds healed, whichever was the sooner.

Data collection

The nurses selecting three layers of graduated Tubigrip were given a questionnaire and asked to report which factors had influenced their choice of selection for each patient. These were related to three categories: patient lifestyle, physical factors and patient factors.

Patient lifestyle

This question sought to explore which lifestyle factors influenced the choice of bandaging system. Three criteria were given:

- the desire by the patient to wear normal footwear
- convenience for the person applying the bandages (this may be the patient, a carer or the nurse)
- 'other' reason.

Physical criteria

This question sought to investigate which physical factors might influence the choice of bandage. Six options were available:

- the need to reduce oedema
- difficulties in mobility
- the presence of infection that required frequent dressing changes
- high levels of exudate that required frequent dressing changes
- large/difficult position of ulcers.
- 'other' reason.

Patient preference

This question sought to investigate how patient preference might influence the nurse in choosing the bandage. Three options were available:

- comfort of the bandages
- cosmetic appearance of the bandages
- 'other' reason.

Patients' experience of using the bandages

Patients were asked to comment on their experience of using three layers of graduated Tubigrip. Specifically, they were asked to comment on:

- the comfort of the bandage
- whether or not it caused irritation to their skin
- whether the bandage stayed in place or slipped down during wear
- whether wearing the bandage interfered with their lifestyle.

Leg ulcer healing

Changes in limb circumference were determined by measuring ankle and calf circumference at the beginning and end of the study. Separate measurements were taken of the ulcer size.

Results

Twenty-eight patients were treated with three layers of graduated Tubigrip; eighteen (64.3%) were female and ten (35.7%) were male. The mean age of patients on entry was 67.9 years (SD=11.9), with a median of 69.5 years (range=50). The mean duration of ulceration before the study was 8.01 months (SD=8.09); the median duration for ulcer duration was 5.5 months (range=29).

Fourteen of the patients' ulcers healed within the twelve-week study period. Of the remaining fourteen patients, a mean reduction in ulcer area of 4.6cm^2 (SD=7.4) was achieved, with a median of 2.3cm^2 (range=28.5).

It is unusual for studies to report the reasons that either patients or nurses give for selecting a bandaging system. This study reports the reasons given by patients and nurses in three domains: lifestyle, physical and patient domains. In addition, nurses were asked to report the most influential factor (if there was one) in selecting this bandaging system.

Nurse choices based on patient lifestyle

The major lifestyle factor that influenced a nurse's decision on bandage choice was the patient's desire to wear shoes (n=19, 67.9%) (*Figure 5.2*). Here, patients requested a bandaging system that was not bulky and would allow them to wear their normal footwear. A further eight (28.6%) patients were selected for this bandage system for the convenience of the person (a nurse, carer or the patient) who was applying the bandage.

Nurse choices based on physical criteria

When considering the physical factors that influenced choice, nurses reported oedema as the primary reason for selecting three layers of graduated Tubigrip (n=12, 42.9%) (*Figure 5.3*). Mobility was the primary reason for ten (35.7%) patients, infection for four (14.3%) patients and the size/position of the ulcer for the remaining two patients (7.1%).

For almost half of these patients, nurses considered the need to reduce oedema as the main physical criteria in choosing this bandaging system. This decision has a sound theoretical basis, as compression is recommended as the mainstay of treatment in patients with venous ulceration and graduated Tubigrip has been shown to provide some degree of compression (Melhuish *et al*, 2000). Mobility was related to footwear and the desire of patients to be able to wear their normal shoes to assist normal mobility. Six patients (21.4%) required frequent dressing changes either because of copious exudate or the presence of infection (prescribed daily topical antiseptic application).

Nurse choices based on patient preference

For the majority of patients (*n*=21, 75.0%) nurses reported that comfort was the factor that influenced their decision to use the three layers of graduated Tubigrip (*Figure 5.4*). A further seven (25.0%) patients reported a range of other factors, including patients wanting to change their own dressings and to participate in the management of their ulcer.

The major influence on nursing in choosing three layers of Tubigrip

Where one factor was considered of overall importance in influencing the decision then this was recorded. Bandage comfort was reported to be the most influential factor for deciding to use three layers of graduated Tubigrip in thirteen (46.4%) patients (*Figure 5.5*). Nurses reported that the convenience of the person applying the bandage was the most influential factor for a further two (7.0%) patients and no one reason was considered more important than another for ten (35.7%) patients. For three patients the 'other' reason was that this system was easy to use.

Who applied the bandages?

The district nurse applied the bandages for seventeen patients, ten patients applied their own bandages and one further patient had a carer applying the bandages (*Figure 5.6*).

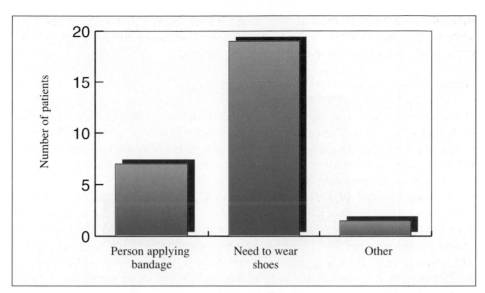

Figure 5.2: Nurse's choice of bandage based on patient lifestyle

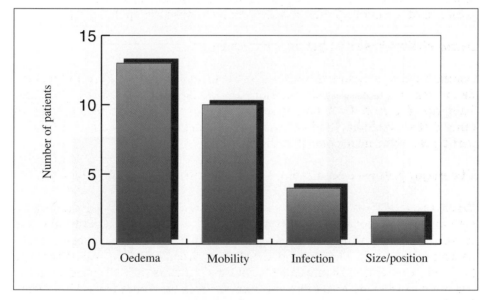

Figure 5.3: Nurse's choice of bandage based on patient's physical criteria

User features of three-layer Tubigrip

This bandaging system performed well in all aspects assessed (*Figure 5.7*). It was rated as being very easy to apply for all twenty-eight patients and a comfortable bandage to wear for twenty-seven (96.4%) patients. In addition, twenty-six (92.9%) patients reported that the bandages stayed in place, were easy to remove, did not irritate their skin and did not interfere with their lifestyle.

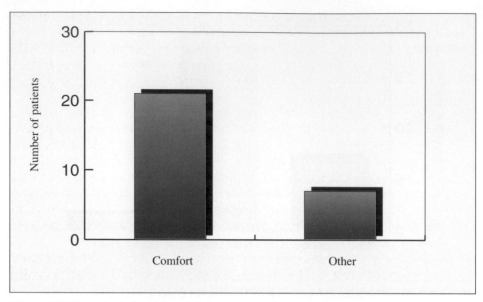

Figure 5.4: Nurse's choice of bandage based on patient's preferences

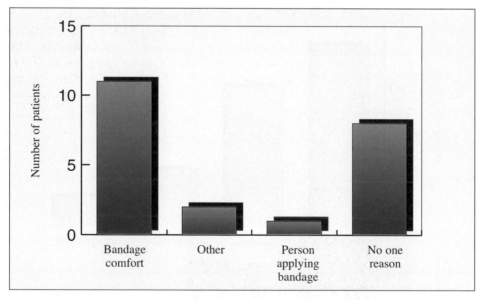

Figure 5.5: The most influential criteria for nurse's choice of bandage

Discussion

Guidelines based on the best evidence are available for managing patients with leg ulceration (Royal College of Nursing Institute, 1998). They provide a structure within which the vast majority of patients can be successfully managed. However, they do not address the issues related to those patients, diagnosed with venous leg ulceration, who cannot tolerate therapeutic compression. These are not a large group of patients, but they do present great challenges to the healthcare professionals caring for them.

When encountering such patients, healthcare professionals are faced with a difficult dilemma: a wide selection of compression treatments are available, but patients decline to accept them, and healthcare professionals must then decide how best to care for them.

It could be argued that conflict exists when the strength of the evidence is counterbalanced by a patient's resistance to the treatments deemed to produce the 'best' outcomes and the patient's agenda differs from that of the nurse. Support for this view comes from Sackett *et al* (1991, 2000) who discuss the role of evidence in clinical decision making. Although they recommend that wherever possible clinical decisions should be based on the best evidence available, they also recognize the complexity of individual patient situations, where it is not always possible for patients to accept the treatment based on best evidence.

In the UK, policy documents recommend that patients become active users of health services (DoH, 1989, 1991, 1999). They also recommend that healthcare professionals work in partnership with patients in making decisions about their treatment. In this study the authors explored the factors that influenced nurses' decisions when they selected a treatment for patients who were unable to tolerate therapeutic compression as the 'best treatment'.

The results suggest that nurses took into account comfort (as the major influence) and lifestyle factors, in addition to efficacy of treatment. This approach is in line with current thinking. Ainsworth and Killingworth (1995), Cahill (1998), the DoH (1999) and Coulter (2000) argue that healthcare professionals should promote patient empowerment and actively seek to involve patients in their own care.

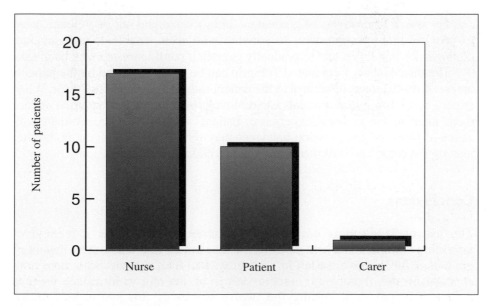

Figure 5.6: Person responsible for applying bandages

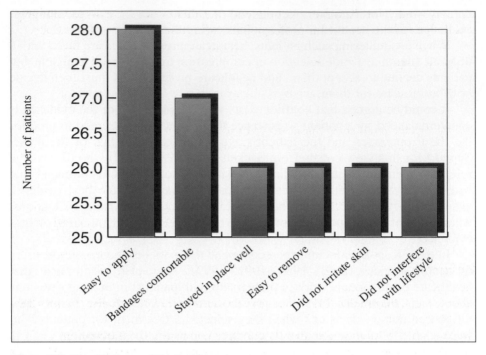

Figure 5.7: User features of the bandage

The most influential factor overall in deciding to use a bandage was patient comfort (see *Figure 5.5*). This is becoming increasingly recognized as problematic for patients with venous leg ulceration (Douglas, 2001). Managing pain has been reported to be a major challenge in treating patients with leg ulceration (Phillips *et al*, 1994; Roe *et al*, 1995; Douglas, 2001).

The use of three layers of graduated Tubigrip emerged out of a clinical need to provide some compression to patients who were unable to use standard compression bandages, and to gradually gain their confidence in using bandages.

The three layers of graduated Tubigrip can be easily removed by the patients and so shifts the locus of control to the patient rather than the nurse/doctor. When experiencing discomfort, patients can remove one of two layers and then replace them later. In the authors' experience, patients unable to be concordant with standard forms of compression bandages may remove them at some point after leaving the clinic and will therefore be left without any compression.

Conclusions

The use of Tubigrip is not recognized or recommended as a method of providing therapeutic levels of compression, but in this study three layers of graduated Tubigrip were used in a novel way to treat patients who were non-concordant with therapeutic compression in an attempt to introduce them to stronger compression. During the twelve weeks of this study, half of the patients' ulcers healed and the remaining patients' ulcers reduced in size. The authors would not, however, recommend that this system was used routinely, but it should be reserved for those patients who have particular difficulties.

Key points

- Not all patients with venous leg ulcers can tolerate high enough levels of compression therapy.
- Nurses in this study considered that patient comfort was the most important factor in selecting a compression bandage for this group of patients.
- Three layers of graduated Tubigrip can be used as an introduction to stronger, therapeutic compression bandages.
- Within a twelve-week period half of patients' ulcers healed, and the remaining fourteen patients experienced a mean reduction in ulcer size of $4.6cm^2$.

References

Ainsworth L, Killingworth A (1995) Tune into your patients' views. *Nurs Manag (Harrow)* **2**(6): 14–15

Bowling A (1997) *Research Methods in Health*. Open University Press, Buckingham

Cahill J (1998) Patient participation: a review of the literature. *J Clin Nurs* **7**(2): 119–28

Closs SJ, Cheater FM (1999) Evidence for nursing practice and a clarification of the issues. *J Adv Nurs* **30:** 10–17

Coulter A (2000) More active role for patients. *Nurs Stand* **14**(45): 5

Department of Health (1989) *Working for Patients*. HMSO, London

Department of Health (1991) *The Patient's Charter*. HMSO, London

Department of Health (1997) *The New NHS: Modern, Dependable*. The Stationery Office, London

Department of Health (1999) *Making a Difference: Strengthening the Nursing, Midwifery and Health Visiting Contribution to Health and Healthcare*. The Stationery Office, London

Doughty DB, Waldrop J, Ramundo J (2000) Lower extremity ulcers of vascular etiology. In: Bryant RA, ed. *Acute and Chronic Wounds*. Mosby, St Louis

Douglas V (2001) Living with a chronic leg ulcer: an insight into patients' experiences and feelings. *J Wound Care* **10**: 355–60

Falanga V (1997) Venous ulceration: assessment, classification and management. In: Krasner D, Kane D, eds. *Chronic Wound Care*. Health Management Publications, Wayne, PA: 165–71

Fletcher A, Cullum N, Sheldon TA (1997) A systematic review of compression treatment for venous leg ulcers. *Br Med J* **315:** 576–80

Haynes B, Haines A (1998) Barriers and bridges to evidence-based practice. (Getting research findings into practice.) *Br Med J* **317:** 273–6

Melhuish J, Wertheim D, Llewellyn M, Williams R, Harding KG (2000) Evaluation of compression under an elastic tubular bandage utilized as an introduction to compression therapy in the treatment of venous leg ulcers. *Phlebology* **15:** 53–9

Moffatt C, Dickson D (1993) The Charing Cross high compression four-layer bandage system. *J Wound Care* **6:** 91–4

Morison M, Moffatt C (1994) Patient assessment. In: *A Colour Guide to the Assessment and Management of Leg Ulcers*. Mosby, London: 33–54

Phillips T, Stanton B, Provan B, Lew RA (1994) A study of the impact of leg ulcers on quality of life: financial, social and psychological implications. *J Am Acad Derm* **31:** 49–53

Roe B, Cullum N, Hamer C (1995) Patients' perceptions of chronic leg ulceration. In: Cullum N, Roe B, eds. *Leg Ulcers: Nursing Management: Research-based Guide*. Scutari, London

Royal College of Nursing Institute (1998) *Clinical Practice Guidelines: The Management of Patients with Leg Ulcers*. RCN Institute, York

Sackett DL, Haynes RB, Guyatt GH, Tugwell P (1991) *Clinical Epidemiology*. Little, Brown, Toronto

Sackett DL, Straus SE, Richardson WS, Rosenberg W, Haynes RB (2000) *Evidence-based Medicine*. Churchill Livingstone, London

Selim P, Lewis C, Templeton S (2001) Evidence-based practice and client compliance. *J Community Nurs* **15**(5): 10–14

Section two:
Wound care: evidence and theory

6

A review of the use of silver in wound care: facts and fallacies

Alan BG Lansdown

This chapter traces the use of silver in wound care, discussing its merits as an antibacterial agent and constituent of many new dressings, which are increasingly tailored to the treatment of wounds ranging from acute surgical lesions to chronic and diabetic leg ulcers. Misconceptions regarding the biological properties of silver, its possible physiological value in the human body and wound bed, absorption through the skin, and safety factors are addressed. The chapter aims to present silver and the new range of sustained silver-release dressings as important features in the management of skin wounds, providing effective control of wound infections while ensuring patient comfort and quality of life.

Silver has made many notable contributions to human health and medicine. In early times, silver coins were used to purify the drinking water of the monarchs of ancient dynasties in the Middle East and South America; since then silver has been employed in prostheses, water purification, surgical needles, catheters, dentistry and wound therapy. Ambrose Paré, the eminent French surgeon (1517–1590), used silver clips in facial reconstruction, and William Halstead (1895), chief surgeon of the Johns Hopkins Medical School, used silver wire sutures in surgery for hernias. Halstead (1895) found that silver foil provided an effective means of dressing surgical wounds and controlling postoperative infection.

Silver nitrate has a history in the treatment of maladies and infectious diseases dating from long before the identification of bacteria, the classic studies of Louis Pasteur and the introduction of Robert Koch's postulates in the 1880s (Evans, 1976; Munch, 2003). Silver nitrate has formed the mainstay of antiseptics used in wound care for more than 150 years, and is still used in burns clinics today.

The antiseptic properties of silver nitrate were appreciated by Credé (1894) who claimed that 0.5–1.0% silver nitrate reduced the incidence of neonatal eye infections in his clinic from 10.8% to about 2%. Early studies indicated that silver nitrate formed 'resistant precipitates' with proteins in skin wounds and that its local antibacterial action could be easily controlled. Lubinsku (1914) remarked that the antiseptic action of silver nitrate extended 'quite deeply' into a wound, with the silver forming soluble double salts of silver albuminate and silver chloride in the tissues.

Silver nitrate is severely caustic at concentrations of 10% or more, but this property is beneficial in the removal of warts, calluses and unsightly granulations (Sollemann, 1942). Nowadays, toughened silver nitrate caustics are licensed by the Medicines Control Agency, but should be used with extreme caution. Surprisingly, Sollemann (1942) remarked that the concentrated solutions of silver nitrate were less painful to patients than the dilute preparations.

Early pharmacologists attempted to overcome the irritancy of silver nitrate by introducing colloidal silver proteins (Sollemann, 1942). They presumed that by precipitating silver in the form of a silver proteinate or colloidal solution, they could overcome the irritancy of free silver ion while preserving its antiseptic action. These colloidal silver proteins achieved some popularity until about thirty years ago, when they were superseded by newer and safer antiseptics, notably penicillins and silver sulphadiazine (now sulfadiazine in the UK) (Lansdown, 2002a).

The introduction of silver sulfadiazine by Fox (1968) marked a renaissance in the use of silver in wound care. While researching the antibiotic therapies available for controlling *Pseudomonas aeruginosa* in burn wounds, Fox noted that two main agents available at the time, dilute silver nitrate solutions and mafenide-containing ointment, were highly effective but had severe disadvantages. Silver nitrate discoloured everything it came into contact with, and caused electrolyte imbalances in wound fluids, while mafenide inhibited key enzymes (eg. carbonic anhydrase) and gave rise to hyperpnoea and hyperchloraemic acidosis.

In introducing silver sulfadiazine, Fox combined the antiseptic properties of silver with sulphonamide, providing a broader spectrum and safer antibiotic for use in wound care and surgery. Fox noted that sulphonamides had been used widely in wound therapy during World War II and were relatively safe. Silver sulfadiazine and silver nitrate have been highly successful in controlling burn wound infections for many years, even though the emergence of sulphonamide-resistant bacteria led to a temporary withdrawal of silver sulfadiazine in some hospitals in the mid-1970s (Lowbury, 1972, 1977; Lowbury *et al*, 1976).

Advances in technology have enabled the manufacturers of wound dressing products to develop safer and more effective antibacterial therapies with barriers to reinfection (Morgan, 1999). The introduction of sustained silver-release dressings in the last twenty years marks a second renaissance in the use of silver in wound therapy. Early dressings included silver-impregnated porcine skin xenografts, silver-impregnated nylon fabrics and meshes and synthetic materials containing silver sulfadiazine for sustained release (Deitch *et al*, 1987; Chu *et al*, 2000). Kawai *et al* (2001) described an artificial dermis based on biodegradable collagen sponge capable of releasing silver sulfadiazine.

Actisorb Silver 220 (Johnson & Johnson) was the first of the modern silver-release dressings to emerge (Mulligan *et al*, 1986; Furr *et al*, 1994). The dressing consists of a carbonized fabric impregnated with metallic silver. Acticoat (Smith and Nephew) was first patented in the USA in 1997 as an antimicrobial coating for medical devices. It was claimed to provide a 'topical, pure silver delivery system' as a burn wound antiseptic (Tredgett *et al*, 1998; Wright *et al*, 1998a; Burrell, 2003).

A variety of silver-release dressings are now licensed in Europe and the USA. They differ greatly in composition, presumed mechanism of action and rate of silver release. They are variously tailored, with recommendations for treating acute surgical wounds, burns and chronic or indolent wounds associated with profound exudation, unpleasant odours and severe patient dis-comfort. All are claimed to be effective against a wide spectrum of bacteria (including methicillin-resistant *Staphylococcus aureus* [MRSA] and vancomycin-resistant enterococci) and to provide an effective barrier to wound re-infection.

Review of the recent literature expounding the merits and clinical advantages of silver-release dressings in wound management reveals factual inaccuracies and misinterpretations, which are perpetuated. These can lead to confusion and uncertainty as to the suitability of silver-release dressings. This chapter attempts to clarify common misconceptions concerning the presumed mechanism of action of silver in the wound bed, its benefits in repair processes, and its relative safety.

Observations on the chemistry of silver

Silver is an inert metal and does not react with human tissues in its non-ionized or 'pure' form. In the presence of moisture, wound fluids and exudates, silver readily ionizes to release Ag^+ or other biologically active ions, which bind with proteins on cell surfaces, including bacteria and fungi. (Silver can form a variety of compounds as Ag^{2+} or Ag^{3+}, but these are rare and unstable.)

Silver is contained in wound dressings in a variety of forms, which vary in their capacity to liberate silver ions. They range from silver metal in microcrystalline form (prepared using nanotechnology, as in Acticoat dressings) and silver-impregnated 'activated' charcoal (Actisorb Silver 220), to inorganic silver compounds such as nitrate, chloride, zirconium lactate, oxide, phosphate, zeolite and sulfadiazine. Organic complexes include colloidal silver preparations, silver proteinates and silver allantoinate. Occasionally, the silver content of a dressing is identified as 'ionic silver or Ag^+' with the identity of the silver complex undefined. Nevertheless, to be effective as an antibacterial/antifungal agent, the silver complex contained in a dressing must release biologically active silver ions.

The solubility and ionization of the silver sources used in wound dressings vary greatly (Burrell, 2003). Silver nitrate is freely soluble and ionizes readily, whereas silver chloride is largely insoluble in water at room temperature and releases only about $1.3\mu g$ Ag+/ml. Gibbons (2003) claimed that an ionic concentration of 1.43ppm (ppm and μg/ml are equivalent) is sufficient to kill or inhibit a wide range of microorganisms. By comparison, products based on microfine particles of silver metal with a particle size of <20nm release 70–100ppm silver ion into a wound site within four hours (Wright *et al*, 1998a; Burrell, 2003). *In vitro* tests have shown that nanocrystalline silver products can maintain antibacterial activity for at least seven days.

Products such as Actisorb Silver 220 utilize a different technology. Silver is adsorbed onto activated charcoal in a high-temperature process, but is not released into the wound site from this dressing (White, 2001). Bacteria are absorbed into the activated charcoal, along with exudates, by a form of wicking, to be killed by ionic silver liberated 'within the dressing' (Scanlon and Dowsett, 2001; Leak, 2002). A similar action is seen with Contreet Foam, which is intended for heavily exudating wounds (Karlsmark *et al*, 2003; Lansdown *et al*, 2003).

Biological properties of silver

Silver is found in minute quantities in the human body ($<2.3\mu$g/litre in blood, urine, liver and kidney) (Wan *et al*, 1991). Higher concentrations might be expected in people exposed to silver or silver dust occupationally. Contrary to statements in the medical literature that silver is a 'trace element' or a 'normal body component', silver has no recognized value as a trace metal nutrient and performs no physiological role in the human body (Lansdown, 1995).

One California-based company even stated that Americans were suffering from the novel and undefined condition of 'silver deficiency'. As far as we know, silver does not accumulate or form reservoirs in any tissue in the body, although there are numerous reports of argyria (deposition of silver salts in the skin) and argyrosis (deposition of silver in the eye) in the literature (Bleehen *et al*, 1981; Lee and Lee, 1994; Lansdown and Williams, 2004).

Argyria usually results from the use of silver nitrate solutions or colloidal silver preparations as oral antiseptics, or from inhalation of silver dust (Pariser, 1978; Bleehen *et al*, 1981). Silver ion absorbed through the intestine or nasal mucosa complexes with blood proteins, to be deposited as silver sulphide or fine granules of silver metal deep in the skin in the region of hair follicles or sweat ducts or in the eye (Bleehen *et al*, 1981). Rarely are true cases of argyria reported following topical application of silver sulfadiazine or silver-containing dressings for skin wounds (Lansdown 2002b, c). Silver is not usually eliminated through the skin, but the dark discolorations fade gradually during tissue remodelling or following normal wear and tear processes.

Colloidal silver preparations were once popular for treating infections ranging from pneumonia, influenza and venereal diseases to bubonic plague and were phased out of pharmacopoeias and national formularies more than thirty years ago for safety reasons (mainly argyria and excessive levels of silver in the blood) (Fung and Bowen, 1996).

A new range of colloidal silver products has emerged in the clandestine market in recent years, with far-fetched claims on the internet and in journals of alternative medicine as to their efficacy as food additives and treatments for AIDs, cancer, infectious diseases, acne, prostatic enlargement and haemorrhoids. These products are claimed to have no known side-effects, but the available evidence is limited and of dubious scientific value (Lansdown, 2002d). Furthermore, it is unlikely that supportive data on these products would meet the stringent regulatory requirements in the UK. Claims that silver released from colloidal silver products acts as a systemic disinfectant and functions like a 'secondary immune system' are complete fantasy.

Silver as an antimicrobial agent

Metal ions can be ranked in order of their antimicrobial activity: silver and mercury head the list and are effective at concentrations of <1ppm *in vitro* (Sykes, 1965). Both metals show an affinity for sulphydryl groups on bacterial cell membranes, and are absorbed into the organisms where they act as cytoplasmic poisons. Von Nägeli is reputed to have coined the expression 'oligodynamic' to describe the lethal effects of metals on susceptible bacteria at concentrations as low as 10–5 to 10–7 silver ions per cell (Romans, 1954).

Early studies (mainly in Germany) suggested that 'active metal ions' are absorbed by bacteria/fungi and coagulate intracellular proteins. Pure metal is inactive. Sensitive organisms accumulate silver from low concentrations in their environment. Silver may have antiviral properties (herpes zoster virus, varicella zoster virus, Herpes virus hominis), but this area is not well documented at present (Chang and Weinstein, 1975; Montes *et al*, 1986).

The bactericidal efficacy of silver ions has been evaluated mainly in *in vitro* culture media (Furr *et al*, 1994; Thomas and McCubbin, 2003a, b). Recent studies using electron microscopy, X-ray microanalysis and enzyme inhibition have provided detailed information on bacterial sensitivity to silver and mechanisms of bactericidal action, and a possible explanation of why certain bacteria are susceptible and others are resistant (Starodub and Trevors, 1989, 1990). Published studies in the past thirty years show that silver absorbed by sensitive strains of organisms such as *Escherichia coli*, *Pseudomonas aeruginosa* and *Klebsiella* species:

- impairs bacterial cell wall integrity
- binds and disrupts subcellular components
- inhibits respiration
- impairs essential enzymes and metabolic events modulated by sodium, magnesium, phosphate, etc.
- inactivates bacterial DNA and RNA.

Bacterial resistance to silver was documented by Lowbury (Lowbury *et al*, 1976; Lowbury, 1977) in clinical trials with silver nitrate and silver sulfadiazine in burns patients at the Birmingham Accident Hospital. Silver sulfadiazine (1%) and a cream containing silver nitrate (0.5%) and 2% chlorhexidine were comparably effective in protecting burns from infection, but silver nitrate compresses were less effective against Gram-negative bacilli. The emergence of sulphonamide-resistant bacilli in extensive burns treated with silver sulfadiazine led to a temporary abandonment of the product. Silver nitrate solution was favoured for treating wounds infected with *Pseudomonas aeruginosa*.

Resistance to silver has been studied in laboratory strains of *Escherichia coli* and *Pseudomonas* species. Starodub and Trevors (1989, 1990) found that silver accumulation by a sensitive strain of E. coli was more than five times higher than that seen in resistant strains. (Sensitive strains of *Klebsiella* accumulated three to four times more silver than did resistant strains.) Silver-sensitive bacteria produced 33% less hydrogen sulphide. Cytochemical and genetic studies (Starodub and Trevors, 1989, 1990) suggest that resistance to silver may be attributable to the formation of silver–sulphide complexes within the cell and intracellular 'protective systems' involving cytoplasmic particles or plasmids. Resistant strains contained two large plasmids (identified as pJT1 and pJT2).

Modern investigative techniques have enabled the molecular and genetic basis for bacterial resistance to silver to be unravelled. Silver and Phung Le (1996) and Gupta *et al* (2001) have cloned and studied the 'determinants' involved in silver resistance in bacteria isolated from burns. They have identified the gene sequences signalling the synthesis of key proteins involved in silver binding or metal uptake in Salmonella species. Further research aims to study environmental and biological causes of bacterial mutagenesis and silver resistance in wounds.

Silver in the wound environment

When a silver-containing dressing is applied to a skin wound, silver ion is released. However, only minute quantities of this free ion penetrate intact human skin because of the effective epidermal barrier function (Coombs *et al*, 1992). When the natural barrier function of the skin is impaired through cuts, lacerations, surgical incisions, burns or ulceration, it can be anticipated that the silver ion liberated from dressings will (Coombs *et al*, 1992):

- be absorbed by bacteria, fungi and inflammatory cells in superficial aspects of the wound
- bind to free sulphydryl groups on/in wound debris
- be absorbed into cells at the wound margin
- penetrate the wound bed
- be absorbed into the systemic circulation.

Although silver can be detected in tissues at concentrations as low as 1ng/L using atomic absorption spectrometry, few clinical or experimental studies are available to illustrate the partition of silver in the different wound compartments (listed above). Even in the most severely infected wounds, only a small proportion of silver entering a wound site will be absorbed by bacteria and be involved in disinfecting the tissues; the remainder will bind with sulphydryl groups and proteins in the wound bed or tissues peripheral to the wound. Studies with silver sulfadiazine suggest that most of the silver absorbed into the body will be excreted via the liver or kidneys (Boosalis *et al*, 1987; Lansdown and Williams, 2004). Measurement of silver in urine or faeces may provide a useful guide to how much silver is absorbed from silver-containing dressings (Boosalis *et al*, 1987). However, the few studies published are inconclusive, either because the concentrations of silver present are very low or because patients exhibit higher than normal background levels of blood silver (argyraemia) as a result of previous medications, silver in food, environmental exposure, etc. (Karlsmark *et al*, 2003).

When a wound is treated with silver nitrate, most silver ion precipitates as black silver sulphide on the surface of wound debris, to be lost as the wound heals. Only minute amounts penetrate the systemic circulation. In contrast, percutaneous uptake of silver sulfadiazine through burns may reach 10%, but uptake tends to be higher in partial-thickness wounds where exposure to severed blood vessels is greater (Coombs *et al*, 1992).

Although Coombs *et al* did not find a clear correlation between silver absorption and burn depth, they noted that serum silver levels were higher in patients with burns extending over larger body areas. At least 50% of the silver absorbed is eliminated within ten to twelve hours, but as much as 45% forms complexes with proteins in wound exudates or the wound bed (Baxter, 1971). It is conceivable that this 'reservoir' of silver will provide a sustained antibacterial action, but little is known about the stability of the complexes or how readily silver is released from them (Dollery, 1991).

Rarely, black discolorations resembling argyria have been reported following the use of silver sulfadiazine or some of the newer dressings releasing high concentrations of silver into the wound site, but the true nature of these deposits awaits analysis (Lansdown and Williams, 2004). A large part of the silver released from silver sulfadiazine and silver-containing dressings that do not leave dark stains in the wound will probably be precipitated as colourless protein complexes in the wound bed. The silver sulfadiazine complex dissociates within the wound, with the sulphonamide moiety being eliminated more rapidly than silver in the urine (Boosalis *et al*, 1987). Silver uptake from wound dressings is not well documented, but is an important area of research that should be addressed as new and highly efficacious silver-containing dressings are accepted into wound care.

Does silver aid wound healing?

Numerous clinical and experimental studies claim that silver released from dressings promotes or kick-starts wound healing by promoting haemostasis, reducing inflammation, and enhancing re-epithelialization and neo-vascularization, but these claims are still the subject of debate (Kjolseth *et al*, 1994; Lansdown *et al*, 1997; Sibbald *et al*, 2000; Karlsmark *et al*, 2003). While acute wounds with low levels of infection and minimal systemic or other complications do seem to heal better in the presence of silver, some chronic or indolent wounds exposed to silver sulfadiazine (Flamazine cream) or silver-containing dressings may persist for many months with questionable signs of improvement (Ballard and McGregor, 2002).

Innes *et al* (2001) do not recommend the use of Acticoat as a dressing for skin graft donor sites. In a recent presentation (Harding, 2003) to the European Tissue Repair Society, Professor Harding remarked on the very high incidence of complications that might impair healing (eg. vascular disease, systemic infections, diabetes, arthritis) in patients with chronic ulcers.

In order to identify ways in which silver might aid wound healing, it may be useful to examine its known action at constituent steps in the so-called wound-healing cascade.

Haemostasis

There do not appear to be any studies which demonstrate that silver released from any product influences haemostasis in acute or chronic skin wounds, even though experimental studies suggest that local calcium concentrations may be raised (calcium is factor IV in blood coagulation) (Lansdown *et al*, 1997). Aquacel Ag is recommended for the treatment of 'wounds that are prone to bleeding' (ConvaTec, 2003), presumably because of the haemostatic properties of the hydrofibre component.

Alginates have been used to aid haemostasis since the 1800s (Blair *et al*, 1990). Avance was claimed to reduce bleeding in a chronic wound in an elderly patient, but the mechanism is not known (Morgan *et al*, 2001).

Inflammation

Equivocal evidence exists to show that silver ion may influence inflammation or granulation tissue formation in skin wounds by a mechanism other than its antibacterial effect. Although clinical trials and case reports frequently note that treatments with Avance, Actisorb Silver 220, Acticoat, Contreet, etc. reduce patient pain and discomfort, this is mostly attributed to the antibacterial effects of the silver and neutralization of the toxins produced by the bacteria, rather than any effects it may have on the infiltration of inflammatory cells into the wound bed.

Demling and DeSanti (2002) claim that meshed autografts promote re-epithelialization in clinical wounds, and refer to the 'prohealing' effects of silver. They attribute this effect to the ability of silver to inhibit the formation of matrix metalloproteinases (MMPs). MMPs tend to be higher in some chronic wounds and may hinder healing. MMPs are mostly zinc-based enzymes involved in the degradation of collagen and wound debris. However, it seems likely that since silver (from Acticoat) encouraged deep burns and ulcers with excessive MMPs to heal, silver can have only a limited propensity to shut off inflammatory changes in a wound site (Demling and DeSanti, 2001, 2002). Experimental studies have demonstrated that suppression of MMPs by topical application of synthetic inhibitors delays healing (Agren *et al*, 2001).

It is of interest to note that the Nucryst Pharmaceuticals division of the Westaim Corporation is currently using nanotechnology to develop a topical silver preparation for the treatment of atopic dermatitis and inflammatory conditions of the skin. Initial pre-clinical studies suggest that the product (NPI32101) has anti-inflammatory properties and broad-spectrum antibacterial activity. Clinical trials are ongoing.

Wound re-epithelialization

More tangible evidence exists to show that, in acute wounds at least, silver can promote cell proliferation and wound healing. Electron microscopy and chemical analysis have shown that silver penetrates living cells at the wound margin, binds to intracellular proteins (including zinc- and copper-binding metallothioneins), and can activate processes that are dependent on metalloenzymes (Lansdown *et al*, 1997; Lansdown, 2002a). Further research is necessary to determine how much silver ion is required to enhance trace metal metabolism in human skin wounds to activate repair processes.

Zinc levels in human skin are six times higher in the epidermis than in the dermis and range from $3-10\mu g/g$ (weight analysis) to about $14-20\mu g/g$ in normally healing wounds and $7-15\mu g/g$ in chronic wounds (Henzel *et al*, 1970). It is conceivable that dressings which release 100ppm silver into the wound within eight to ten hours (Wright *et al*, 1998a,b) will significantly enhance zinc or copper levels to trigger or kick-start wound repair, as claimed in product information documents, but clinical evidence is urgently required.

It will be interesting to see whether silver influences other features in the wound environment to advance chemotactic pathways, cell migration patterns and maturation, which are critical during the later stages of wound reorganization and normalization.

Preclinical evaluation of silver products in wound care

Laboratory studies form an essential preclinical step in the development of any medicine or healthcare product. A sequence of meticulously controlled tests are conducted under defined conditions to assess the physicochemical characteristics of a product, its stability, release of bioactive constituents, pharmacological properties and potential toxicity.

In the case of silver, microbiological tests are a major component of the preclinical evaluation (Furr *et al*, 1994; Bowler *et al*, 1998). Tests will be conducted *in vitro* to identify the minimum concentrations necessary to kill or inhibit 50% of named organisms (including bacteria or fungi isolated from human wounds) and other features of their bactericidal profile (Furr *et al*, 1994; Thomas and McCubbin, 2003a, b). Preclinical studies provide a cost-effective means of determining which products are suitable for clinical trials and which should be abandoned.

Tissue and cell culture techniques are now sufficiently advanced to allow any cell type in the human body to be cultured under defined conditions of culture medium, temperature, oxygen, etc. Keratinocytes, fibroblasts, neutrophils and macrophages can be shown to respond to growth factors, nutrients, cytokines, hormones and other factors that influence proliferation, migration and maturation in an intact tissue. Cells can be cultured to provide multilaminate structures resembling the epidermis, with evidence of cell and biochemical gradients representing *in vivo* tissue physiology.

Cell culture techniques have been used to examine the toxicity of silver and to identify the minimum toxic dose (Hidalgo *et al*, 1998; Gibbons, 2003). However, none of these systems can adequately reproduce the complex environment present in any repairing or regenerating tissue *in situ*. The skin exists naturally in a state of dynamic equilibrium with its environment and exhibits a defined and genetically determined programme of cell death and regeneration in response to normal wear and tear and injury.

Modulation of the processes involved is highly complex and incompletely understood. Only limited success has been achieved so far in understanding the complex chemical and nutrient gradients involved in cell migration and maturation, the nutritional requirements, and the role of hormones, growth factors and conditions in the microenvironment.

Cultured cells are to all intents 'naked cells'. They are highly vulnerable to physical and chemical conditions in the local environment. Hidalgo *et al* (1998) demonstrated that cultured fibroblasts are sensitive to silver nitrate concentrations 100–700 times lower than those required to disinfect skin wounds in clinical practice. It is unrealistic to predict that a concentration of silver capable of killing 50% of cells in culture (IC50) will produce evidence of skin toxicity when applied to a wound. If the results of titrating silver against mammalian cell cultures showing an IC50 of 50ppm in twenty-four hours were to be extrapolated to a chronic wound situation, dressings releasing 100ppm silver would clearly be unacceptable. Experience has shown that Acticoat 7 and Contreet Foam are effective products for wound care and are without toxic risk (Demling and DeSanti, 2001; Karlsmark *et al*, 2003). The results of *in vitro* tests should always be viewed with extreme caution (Lansdown and Williams, 2004).

Laboratory animal studies have a part to play in investigating the possible benefits of silver-containing products on wound repair and regeneration, and their possible mechanisms of action. Although they can provide a satisfactory means of predicting the toxicity of drugs, medicaments and devices used in human medicine, they should also be extrapolated with care (Lansdown, 1978, 1995; Meyer *et al*, 1978).

Human skin is unique in the animal kingdom and has no exact counterpart, even among higher primates (Kligman, 1978). No animal model can provide other than preliminary information that a product is potentially useful and safe for use in wound care, or that product A is better than B or worse than C. While cell proliferation patterns, migratory pathways and maturation are likely to be similar in experimental and human wounds, it is important to recognize that there are fundamental interspecies differences (*Table 6.1*).

Toxicity of silver in medicine

Accurate information on the toxicity of silver is hard to find. What does exist is frequently fragmentary, occasionally misleading or incompletely evaluated.

Silver is absorbed into the human body through the intestinal mucosa, by inhalation and through skin wounds. The silver ion is highly reactive and shows an affinity for sulphydryl (SH) groups on cell membranes and proteins in a wound or in the circulation. Silver protein complexes are formed in the systemic circulation and can be mobilized to and deposited in any organ or tissue in the body — particularly the skin, liver, kidneys, bone marrow and eyes. The available evidence shows that although silver can cause transitory changes, including leucopenia, the risk of lasting damage or persistent functional disorder in any tissue is very low (Lansdown and Williams, 2004). Silver is eliminated in the urine and faeces, but little is currently known about the patterns of silver metabolism from deposits in any organ. It is not known to what extent silver accumulates in bone or hard tissue.

Allergy to silver is associated with occupational exposure (eg. silver worker's finger) and silver in jewellery (Fisher, 1987). The extent to which silver allergy arises in the use of silver-containing wound dressings is not known, but manufacturers normally warn customers of this potential risk.

Patients with chronic wounds do occasionally experience discomfort with silver-containing dressings. Although silver allergy might be diagnosed, the possibility that the patient is sensitive to other materials in the dressing or the environment should not be discounted. Some patients have particularly sensitive skin contraindicating the use of all but the blandest of dressings. Lanolin, paraffin wax, antibiotics (other than silver), antihistamines, latex gloves, and glove powder are all well known causes of skin reactions and delayed hypersensitivity (Fisher, 1987). Hyperthermia, excessive dehydration and reduced gas permeability of a dressing may be contributory factors.

Table 6.1: Interspecies differences in relation to wounds
All wounds induced in the skin of experiemtnal animals are of the acute type; chronic wounds cannot be induced in non-human species
Animal skin wounds are usually induced in genetically defined animals maintained under critically controlled laboratory conditions
The natural flora of animal skin differs from that of human skin
The immunological reactivity of animal skin differs from that of human skin (Marzulli *et al*, 1968; Kligman, 1978)
No non-human species can accurately reproduce the wide diversity of human skin types, which vary according to race, sex, genotype, diet and geographical area
The constitution of epidermal lipids, sweat gland secretions and epidermal barrier are species specific
It is difficult or impossible to reproduce clinical symptoms of human diseases that influence wound healing in human patients, eg. diabetes mellitus

Conclusion

The ability of silver ion to kill or otherwise inhibit a wide range of Gram-positive and Gram-negative bacteria, filamentous fungi and some viruses found in skin wounds is unequivocal. Silver is effective at low concentrations and, with the exception of occasional incidences of contact allergy (delayed hypersensitivity), is without appreciable toxic risk.

Modern technology and improved understanding of the pathology and cytological behaviour of the wound bed have led to the introduction of a new generation of silver-containing dressings for wound care. These dressings are realistically tailored to the treatment of specific wound types, ranging from acute surgical lesions to burns, chronic leg ulcers and diabetic ulcers, some of which are notoriously prone to infection.

There is good evidence that infections are a major cause of chronicity and failure in wound healing, but clinical observations show that chronic wounds are frequently complicated by vascular disease, arthritis, diabetes mellitus and systemic infections. Although silver is frequently able to control wound infections or provide an effective barrier to re-infection, drugs or other therapy given to treat these other conditions may counteract any beneficial influence of silver on or in the wound bed.

The silver-release dressings introduced in recent years use metallic silver, inorganic silver compounds and organic complexes as their source of silver, and components such as polyurethane, alginates, carboxymethylcellulose, knitted fabrics and activated charcoal provide the structure of the dressing. The dressings vary greatly in their total silver content (from 1.6 to $546mg/100cm^2$), capacity to release free silver ion, and presumed depth of silver penetration into the wound.

Dressings are designed in different ways to modulate silver-release patterns. Selection of an appropriate dressing will invariably be a subjective decision based on the personal judgment and experience of clinicians or tissue viability nurses, aided by advice from manufacturers. Questions do arise for which there are no ready answers. A common question is how much silver is sufficient to treat a wound without producing undesirable side-effects. Answers to these and other questions, with explanations, may become available as more experience is gained and research studies are completed.

Laboratory tests are an essential first step in the development of any medicament, but however meticulously they are conducted in a test tube, tissue culture system or laboratory animal model, they cannot realistically represent conditions in the human wound. Routine microbiological tests have a place in identifying the susceptibility of infectious agents (type cultures or wound isolates) to ionized silver released from a dressing, and may prove useful in comparing the antimicrobial efficacy of different dressings (Wright *et al*, 1998a, b; Thomas and McCubbin, 2003a, b). Preclinical research studies are designed to predict how a medicament or dressing might behave in a clinical situation, but they can at best only provide an approximate guide to nurses or clinicians.

Although the value of silver in wound care has been appreciated for many years, research still has a major place in providing answers to the questions that regularly arise in clinical and manufacturing practice. We need to use appropriate hospital resources (eg. clinical chemistry, biopsy pathology, haematology and sonography) to investigate how a wound responds to a particular silver dressing, where the silver goes (ie. its distribution between wound infections, wound exudate proteins, wound bed, etc.) and rates of elimination of silver from the wound site.

Despite earlier reports indicating hazards with silver nitrate, colloidal silver and metallic silver (Rungby, 1990; Fung and Bowen, 1996; Humphries and Routledge, 1998), minimal evidence has been found to suggest that silver is toxic when released into the wound, even at high concentrations (Hollinger, 1996; Lansdown and Williams, 2004).

Argyria is a possible side-effect of the use of silver or silver-containing dressings, but this is cosmetic, usually only temporary and not life-threatening. Research is necessary to investigate the condition colloquially known as 'silver dumping'. Chemical analysis may prove useful in identifying the nature of the dark-coloured deposits seen occasionally in patients with heavily exudating wounds treated with high-silver dressings.

It is to be hoped that careful analysis and thoughtful information from laboratory and clinical research will provide a clearer understanding of the importance of silver in wound care, and help to distinguish the facts from the fiction.

The author would like to thank the staff of the Department of Venous Surgery at Charing Cross Hospital, London, for their guidance and helpful advice.

Key points

⌘ Silver is a broad-spectrum antibacterial and antifungal agent with limited antiviral properties. It has no role in the body as a trace metal nutrient.

⌘ Silver is available as a topical antiseptic (silver nitrate or silver sulphadiazine) and as an anti-infective agent in wound dressings at concentrations ranging from 1.6 to 500mg/ 100cm^2, with widely varying patterns of silver ion release.

⌘ Silver-containing dressings are tailored to the treatment of wounds ranging from acute surgical lesions with low-grade infections to chronic indolent and diabetic wounds and ulcers with recurrent infections, exudation and odour.

⌘ Silver-containing dressings are designed for easy application, maximal patient comfort and safety in use. They provide a barrier to common pathogens.

⌘ Further research and clinical observation is needed to establish how much silver is necessary to eliminate infections in chronic wounds and provide an effective barrier function.

References

Agren MS, Mirastschijski U, Karlsmark T, Saarialho-Kere UK (2001) Topical synthetic inhibitor of matrix metallo-proteinases delays epidermal regeneration in human wounds. *Exp Dermatol* **10**: 337–48

Ballard K, McGregor F (2002) Avance: silver hydropolymer dressing for critically colonized wounds. *Br J Nurs* **11**: 206–11

Baxter CL (1971) Topical use of 1% silver sulphadiazine. In: Polk HC, Stone H, eds. *Contemporary Burn Management*. Little, Brown & Co, Boston: 217–25

Blair SD, Jarvis P, Salmon M, McCollum CN (1990) Clinical trial of calcium alginate haemostatic swabs. *Br J Surg* **77**: 568–70

Bleehen SS, Gould DJ, Harrington CI, Durrant TE, Slater DN, Underwood JC (1981) Occupational argyria: light and electron-microscopic studies and X-ray microanalysis. *Br J Dermatol* **104**: 19–26

Boosalis MG, McCall JT, Ahrenholz DH, Solem LD, McClain CT (1987) Serum and urinary silver levels in thermal injury patients. *Surgery* **101**: 40–3

Bowler PG, Jones SA, Davies BJ, Coyle E (1998) Infection control of some wound dressings. *J Wound Care* **8**: 499–502

Burrell RE (2003) A scientific perspective on the use of topical silver preparations. *Ostomy Wound Manage* **49**(Suppl 5A): 19–24

Chang TW, Weinstein L (1975) In vitro activity of silver sulphadiazine against herpes virus hominis. *J Infect Dis* **132**: 79–81

Chu CS, Matylevitch NP, McManus AT, Goodwin CW, Pruitt BA (2000) Accelerated healing with a mesh autograft/allodermal composite skin graft treated with silver nylon dressings with and without direct current in rats. *J Trauma* **49**: 115–25

ConvaTec (2003) *ConvaTec Technical Data Sheet: Aquace*l. ConvaTec, Uxbridge

Coombs CJ, Wan AT, Masterton JP, Conyers RA, Pedersen J, Chia YT (1992) Do burns patients have a silver lining? *Burns* **28**: 179–84

Credé KSF (1894) *Die verhutung der argentzundung der neugeborenen der haufigsten und wuchtigsten ursache der blindheit.* Ed. A Hirschwald

Deitch EA, Marino AA, Malenkok V, Albright JA (1987) Silver nylon cloth in vitro and in vivo evaluation of antimicrobial activity. *J Trauma* **27**: 301–14

Demling RH, DeSanti L (2001) Effects of silver on wound management. *Wounds: A Compendium of Clinical Research and Practice* **13**(Suppl A): 4–15

Demling RH, DeSanti L (2002) The rate of re-epithelialization across meshed skin grafts is increased with exposure to silver. *Burns* **28**: 264–6

Dollery CL (1991) Silver sulphadiazine. *Current Therapeutic Drugs* **2**: 6

Evans AS (1976) Causation and disease: the Henle-Koch postulates revisited. *Yale J Biol Med* **49**: 175–95

Fisher AA (1987) *Contact Dermatitis.* 3rd edn. Lea and Febiger, Philadelphia

Fox CL (1968) Silver sulfadiazine: a new topical therapy for *Pseudomonas* in burns. Theory of *Pseudomonas* infection in burns. *Arch Surg* **96**: 184–8

Fung MC, Bowen DL (1996) Silver products for medical indications: risk–benefit assessment. *Clin Toxicol* **34**: 119–26

Furr JR, Russell AD, Turner AD, Andrews A (1994) Antibacterial activity of Actisorb Plus, Actisorb and silver nitrate. *J Hosp Infect* **27**: 201–8

Gibbons BL (2003) How Much is too Much Silver? Abstract. Wounds UK 2003, Harrogate, 11–12 November

Gupta A, Phung Le T, Taylor DE, Silver S (2001) Diversity of silver resistance in IncH incompatability plasmids. *Microbiology* **147**: 3393–402

Halstead WS (1895) The operative treatment of hernia. *JAMA* **110**: 13–17

Harding KG (2003) *13th Annual Meeting of the European Tissue Repair Society.* De Meervaart, Amsterdam, the Netherlands

Henzel JH, DeWeese MS, Lichti EL (1970) Zinc concentrations within healing wounds. Significance of postoperative zincuria on availability and requirements during tissue repair. *Arch Surg* **100**: 349–57

Hidalgo E, Bartolome R, Barroso C, Moreno A, Dominguez C (1998) Silver nitrate: antimicrobial activity related to cytotoxicity in cultured human fibroblasts. *Skin Pharmacol Appl Skin Physiol* **11**: 140–51

Hollinger MA (1996) Toxicological aspects of silver pharmaceuticals. *Crit Rev Toxicol* **26**: 255–60

Humphries SDM, Routledge PA (1998) The toxicology of silver nitrate. *Adverse Drug Reactions Toxicology Review* **12**: 115–43

Innes ME, Umraw N, Fish JS, Gomez M, Cartotto RC (2001) The use of silver-coated dressings on donor site wounds: a prospective, controlled matched pair study. *Burns* **27**: 621–7

Karlsmark T, Agerslev RH, Bendz SH, Larsen JR, Roed-Petersen J, Andersen KE (2003) Clinical performance of a new silver dressing, Contreet Foam, for chronic exuding venous leg ulcers. *J Wound Care* **12**: 351–4

Kawai K, Suzuki S, Tabata Y, Taira T, Ikada Y, Nishimura Y (2001) Development of an artificial dermis preparation capable of silver sulphadiazine release. *J Biomed Mater Res* **57**: 346–56

Kjolseth D, Frank DM, Barker JH et al (1994) Comparison of the effects of commonly used wound agents on epithelialization and neo-vascularization. *J Am Coll Surg* **179**: 305–12

Kligman AM (1978) Cutaneous toxicology: an overview from the underside. *Curr Probl Dermatol* **7**: 1–25

Lansdown ABG (1978) Animal models for the study of skin irritants. *Curr Probl Dermatol* **7**: 26–38

Lansdown ABG (1995) Physiological and toxicological changes in the skin resulting from the action and interaction of metal ions. *Crit Rev Toxicol* **25**: 397–462

Lansdown ABG (2002a) Metallothioneins: potential therapeutic aids for wound healing in the skin. *Wound Repair Regen* **10**: 130–2

Lansdown ABG (2002b) Silver 1: its antibacterial properties and mechanism of action. *J Wound Care* **11**: 125–30

Lansdown ABG (2002c) Silver 2: toxicity in mammals and how its products aid wound repair. *J Wound Care* **11**: 173–7

Lansdown ABG (2002d) Controversies over colloidal silver. *J Wound Care* **12**: 120

Lansdown ABG, Williams A (2004) How safe is silver in wound care? *J Wound Care* **13**(4): 1–7

Lansdown ABG, Sampson B, Laupattarakasem P, Vuttivirojana A (1997) Silver aids healing in the sterile wound: experimental studies in the laboratory rat. *Br J Dermatol* **137**: 728–35

Lansdown ABG, Jensen K, Jensen M (2003) Contreet Foam and Contreet Hydrocolloid: an insight into two new silver-containing dressings. *J Wound Care* **12**: 205–10

Leak K (2002) PEG site infections: a novel use for Actisorb Silver 220. *Br J Community Nurs* **7**: 321–5

Lee SM, Lee SH (1994) Generalized argyria after habitual use of silver nitrate. *J Dermatol* **21**: 50–3

Lowbury EJL (1972) Special problems in hospital antisepsis. In: Russell AD, Hugo WB, Ayliff GAJ, eds. *Principles and Practice of Disinfection, Preservation and Sterilization.* Blackwell Scientific, Oxford: 310–29

Lowbury EJL (1977) Problems of resistance in open wounds and burns. In: Mouton RP, Brumfitt W, Hamilton-Miller JMT, eds. *The Rational Choice of Antibacterial Agents.* Kluwer Harrap, London: 18–31

Lowbury EJL, Babb JR, Bridges K, Jackson DM (1976) Topical chemoprophylaxis with silver sulphadiazine and silver nitrate-chlorhexidine creams: the emergence of sulphonamide-resistant Gram-negative bacilli. *Br Med J* **i**: 493–6

Lubinsku W (1914) Silbernitrat oder Silberweiss. *Berlin Klin Wchnschr* **51**: 1643

Marzulli FN, Carson T, Maibach HI (1968) *Delayed hypersensitivity studies in man and animals. Proceedings of the Joint Conference on Cosmetic Science.* The Toilet Goods Association, Washington DC

Meyer W, Schwartz R, Neurand K (1978) The skin of domestic mammals as a model for human skin with special reference to the domestic pig. *Curr Probl Dermatol* **7**: 39–52

Montes LF, Muchinik G, Fox CL (1986) Host responses to varicella zoster virus and herpes zoster virus to silver sulphadiazine. *Cutis* **38**: 363–5

Morgan DA (1999) Wound management products in the Drug Tariff. *The Pharmaceutical Journal* **263**: 820–5

Morgan T, Evans C, Harding KG (2001) A study to measure patient comfort and acceptance of Avance™, a new polyurethane foam dressing containing silver and antimicrobial when used to treat chronic wounds. Presented at the 11th European Wound Management Association Meeting, Dublin

Mulligan CM, Bragg AJ, O'Toole OB (1986) A controlled comparative trial of Actisorb activated charcoal cloth dressings in the community. *Br J Clin Pract* **40**(4): 145–8

Munch R (2003) Robert Koch. *Microbes Infect* **5**(1): 69–74

Pariser RJ (1978) Generalized argyria: clinico-pathological features and histochemical studies. *Arch Dermatol* **114**: 373–7

Romans IB (1954) *Antiseptics, Disinfectants, Fungicides and Chemical and Physical Sterilization.* Kimpton, London

Rungby J (1990) An experimental study on silver in the nervous system and on aspects of its general cellular toxicity. *Dan Med Bull* **37**: 442–9

Scanlon L, Dowsett C (2001) Clinical governance in the control of wound infection and odour. *Br J Nurs* **10**(Silver Suppl Pt 2): 9–18

Sibbald RG, Coutts P, Browne A, Coehlo S (2000) *Acticoat, a new ionised silver-coated dressing: its effect on bacterial load and healing rates*. Wound Healing Society Educational Programme, Toronto, Canada

Silver S, Phung Le T (1996) Bacterial heavy metals resistance; new surprises. *Annu Rev Microbiol* **50**: 753–89

Sollemann T (1942) *A Manual of Pharmacology*. 6th edn. Saunders, Philadelphia: 1102–9

Starodub ME, Trevors JT (1989) Silver resistance in *Escherichia coli* R1. *J Med Microbiol* **29**: 101–10

Starodub ME, Trevors JT (1990) Silver accumulation and resistance in Escherichia coli R1. *J Inorg Biochem* **39**: 317–25

Sykes G (1965) *Disinfection and Sterilization Theory and Practice*. 2nd edn. E & FN Spon, London: 418–22

Thomas S, McCubbin P (2003a) A comparison of the antimicrobial effects of four silver-containing dressings on three organisms. *J Wound Care* **12**: 1011–107

Thomas S, McCubbin P (2003b) An in vitro analysis of the antimicrobial properties of 10 silver-containing dressings. *J Wound Care* **12**: 305–8

Tredgett EE, Shankowski HA, Groenveld A, Burrell RE (1998) A matched pair, randomized study evaluating the efficacy and safety of Acticoat silver-coated dressing for the treatment of burn wounds. *J Burn Care Rehabil* **19**: 531–7

Wan AT, Conyers RA, Coombs CJ, Masterton JP (1991) Determination of silver in blood, urine and tissues of volunteers and burn patients. *Clin Chem* **37**: 1683–7

White RJ (2001) A charcoal dressing with silver in wound infection: clinical evidence. *Br J Nurs* **10**(Silver Suppl Pt 2): 4–8

Wright JB, Hansen DL, Burrell RE (1998a) The comparative efficacy of two antimicrobial barrier dressings: in vitro examination of two controlled release silver dressings. *Wounds: A Compendium of Clinical Research and Practice* **10**: 179–88

Wright JB, Lam K, Burrell RE (1998b) Wound management in an era of increasing bacterial resistance. A role for topical silver. *Am J Infect Control* **26**: 572–7

7

Criteria for wound infection by indication

Keith F Cutting, Richard J White

Clinical criteria for the identification of wound infection are regularly based on a list created by Cutting and Harding (1994). This list was established from empirical data generated in a large, multidisciplinary clinical practice, and is now widely accepted as a seminal article in wound care. Both Cutting (1998) and Gardner *et al* (2001) have conducted validation exercises on these wound infection criteria, based on the assumption that the criteria broadly apply to most wound types. Although many of the original criteria do apply across the spectrum of wound types, the major categories of wounds should be considered separately to avoid the possibility of overlooking the presence of infection. The focus of this chapter is a review of the published literature on wound infection criteria for acute and surgical wounds, diabetic foot ulcers, venous and arterial leg ulcers, pressure ulcers and burns. All known criteria for each wound type are presented, as well as an outline of the ongoing research project to refine the criteria by wound type using a Delphi panel technique. No attempt has been made to correlate visual signs and symptoms with microbiological sampling techniques. It is clear that there are subtle variations between infection criteria for wound types and that these should be recognized if treatment is to be given appropriately and promptly, and morbidity avoided.

The accurate identification of wound infection is a challenge for any clinician involved in this area of care and can have a significant impact on patient morbidity. The more obvious signs such as purulent discharge and spreading erythema are recognized as diagnostic of established wound infection. However, these features are not always present in the early stages when diagnosis is important for treatment and the avoidance of complicating sequelae.

There are additional subtle signs (clinical indicators) that herald the onset of infection. Following a review of the available literature, Cutting and Harding (1994) attempted to collate the indicators of infection. The aim was to include all clinical indicators of acute and chronic wound infection that had been used by colleagues in the field and had been shown to be of value, either by being generated through research or through empirical findings. These collated criteria appear to have gained acceptance not only in the UK but also overseas.

The Cutting and Harding (1994) criteria (*Table 7.1*) brought to the attention of many clinicians subtle criteria that may not have previously been considered, or that had eluded their own exploration of the subject matter. For an explanation of the subtle nature of the additional criteria, the reader is referred to the original paper (Cutting and Harding, 1994).

These criteria provide a reminder or checklist and it is likely that many clinicians have put the criteria to the test in their own clinical practices. For any clinical tool to be of proven value it needs to be tested and there have been two validation studies challenging the Cutting and Harding criteria (1994); these are Cutting (1998) and Gardner *et al* (2001).

Cutting (1998) tested the criteria by asking ward nurses to view patients' wounds and to make a decision on the infection status of the wound by using their own criteria. These decisions were then compared with the researcher's verdict, using the Cutting and Harding (1994) criteria, and a microbial assay of the wound taken via wound swab. A consultant microbiologist also took decisions on the infection status of the wound from results of the cultures.

Table 7.1: Criteria for identifying wound infection
Traditional wound infection criteria
• Abscess
• Cellulitis
• Discharge, including; serous exudate with inflammation, seropurulent, haemopurulent and pus
Additional criteria
• Delayed healing
• Discoloration
• Friable granulation tissue which bleeds easily
• Unexpected pain or tenderness
• Pocketing at the base of the wound
• Bridging of the epithelium or soft tissue (*Figure 7.1*)
• Abnormal smell

Cutting and Harding, 1994

A total of twenty nurses took part in the study. Two nurses at a time viewed four wounds, so a total of forty different patients' wounds were seen which allowed eighty opportunities for separate decisions to be made. Although the types of wounds included in the study were not made explicit in the publication, all of the wounds were healing by secondary intention and did not include burns or leg ulcers. The findings in this study (Cutting, 1998) indicated that the criteria have a high degree of validity. Thirty-nine of the forty decisions (97.5%) made by the researcher on the infected status of the wounds were corroborated by the wound swab culture.

Gardner *et al* (2001) examined the validity of the classic signs of infection (pain, erythema, oedema, heat and purulence) and,

... signs specific to secondary intention wounds (ie. serous exudate, delayed healing, discolouration of granulation tissue, friable granulation tissue, pocketing at the base of the wound, foul odour and wound breakdown).

The wound types against which the criteria were tested were described in the study as 'a mix of chronic wounds,' and subjects were enrolled who had a 'non-arterial chronic wound'. These types of wounds are defined as,

... wounds caused by prolonged pressure, venous insufficiency, peripheral neuropathy, surgical incision (healing by secondary intention) or trauma.

It is also important to note that one of the criteria included by Cutting and Harding (1994) — 'bridging of the epithelium or soft tissue' – was omitted from the clinical signs and symptoms checklist (CSSC) used in this study (*Figure 7.1*). No explanation for this is given by Gardner *et al* (2001). The list of twelve features included in CSSC is presented in *Table 7.2*.

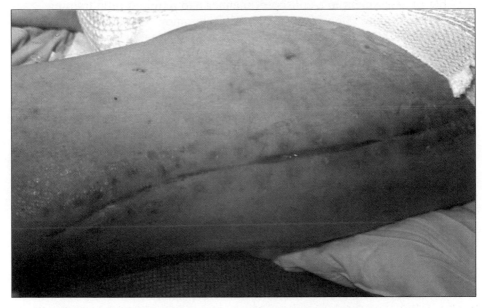

Figure 7.1: Bridging of the epithelium in a primary surgical wound

The results show that the signs specific to secondary wounds are more accurate as indicators of infection than the classic signs. The only sign that did not demonstrate validity was pocketing of the wound base. This is an unexpected finding as pocketing at the base of the wound was found by Marks *et al* (1985) to be indicative of deficient granulation tissue due to an uneradicated infection, and therefore diagnostic of infection in pilonidal sinus excisions left to heal by secondary intention. To the authors' knowledge, this feature (pocketing at the base of a wound) has not been observed or reported as an indicator of infection in a pressure ulcer or ulcer of the lower limb. The signs showing validity (based on the four parameters of sensitivity, specificity, discriminatory power and positive predictive value) were increasing

Table 7.2: Clinical signs and symptoms checklist
• Increasing pain in the wound area
• Erythema
• Oedema
• Heat
• Purulent exudate
• Serous exudate
• Delayed healing of the wound
• Discolouration of the granulation tissue
• Pocketing at the base of the wound
• Foul odour
• Wound breakdown

Gardner *et al*, 2001

wound pain, friable granulation tissue, foul odour and wound breakdown.

Cutting and Harding (1994) produced a set of objective and subjective criteria to help identify wound infection. While criteria that are subjective in nature are thought to be of limited value, Gardner *et al* (2001) found that the inter-rater reliability of the subjective elements (touch, colour and smell) were capable of assessment in a consistent manner and required little training.

Although most infected wounds exhibit common 'classical' criteria, there are subtle differences between wound types. A weakness of Cutting and Harding (1994) was that the original set of criteria developed did not differentiate between different wound types. This was because of a failure to recognize that diverse wound types could exhibit different criteria. It is interesting to note that this tenet appears to have been omitted from a joint consensus meeting of the European Tissue Repair Society and the European Wound Management Association considering chronic wound infection (Leaper, 1998). Focus on different wound types is now considered to be essential so that these understated and possibly misunderstood variations are recognized, enabling accurate identification of infection.

The following sets of criteria have been developed using a similar process to Cutting and Harding (1994). The literature has been reviewed and, where possible, criteria deemed to be indicative of infection in a particular wound type have been generated. The purpose of this exercise is to draw attention to the variations in criteria that may occur for different wound types. There is undoubtedly some overlap between groups and if this were not the case, the Cutting and Harding (1994) criteria would have been of limited benefit in the intervening years. Reviewing the literature to assist in identifying infection in fungating wounds was not pursued. These lesions present enormous challenges to the clinician and the effects of the underlying pathology on the tissues results in devitalized tissue and polymicrobial activity, the effects of which are almost impossible to determine. To assist the reader the criteria are presented in a tabular format with the relevant references.

Diabetic foot ulcers

Foot ulceration and infection are major causes of hospitalization in people with diabetes (Boulton and Bowker, 1985). Signs of infection in these lesions are likely to be 'masked' as people with diabetes may not show typical inflammatory response to infection (pain, erythema, swelling and leucocytosis). Despite this inherent difficulty, diagnosis of infection is essentially clinical (Armstrong *et al*, 1996). In addition, infection of the diabetic foot often involves superficial and deep tissues, including bone. This is unlike other common chronic wound types and will accordingly manifest in different criteria for infection (*Table 7.3*) (*Figure 7.2*).

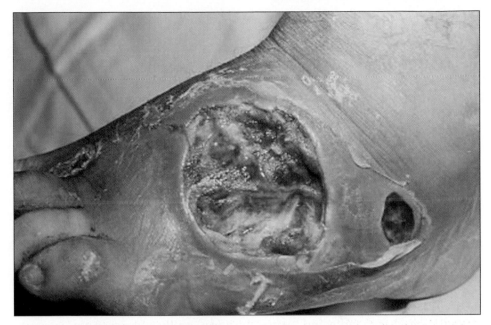

Figure 7.2: Infected diabetic foot ulcer

Table 7.3: Signs of infection of diabetic foot lesions

presence of two
suggests infection[1]

- Heat swelling[1]
- Erythema[1]
- Lymphangitis[1]
- Foul smell[1] (NB no odour if infected with *staphylococci* or *streptococci*)
- Induration[1]
- Fever and other systemic signs[1]
- Pain[1]

- Crepitus with cellulitis[2]
- Sinus tract formation[3]
- Osteomyelitis[1]
- Cellulitis
- Probing to bone[1,4]

1. Edmonds M (2002) Ulcer research classification consensus meeting. *The Diabetic Foot* **5**(1): 12–14
2. Sapico F, Bessman A (1991) Diabetic foot infections. In: Fryberg R, ed. *The High Risk Foot in Diabetes Mellitus*. Churchill Livingstone, New York
3. Caputo GM, Cavanagh PR, Ulbrecht JS, Gibbons GW, Karchmer AW (1994) Assessment and management of foot disease in patients with diabetes. *N Engl J Med* **331**(13): 854–60
4. Grayson Gibbons GW, Balogh K, Levin E, Karchmer AW (1995) Probing to bone in infected pedal ulcers: a clinical sign of underlying osteomyelitis in diabetic patients. *JAMA* **273**: 721–3

Pressure ulcers

Heggers (1998) suggested that pressure ulcers may not only become infected but that infection may be implicated in aetiology. The rationale for this is that the localization of pressure encourages bacterial concentration in that area and bacterial enzymes and toxins (Cooper, 2003) precipitate loss of superficial skin.

The identification of wound malodour is reliant on the individual's acuity of smell (Cutting and Harding, 1994) and depends on the microbial species present (Bowler *et al*, 1999). Anaerobes are traditionally linked to malodour but the influence of aerobic or anaerobic synergy should not be ruled out as a cause of malodour, particularly when Gram-negative anaerobes are involved (Bowler *et al*, 1999).

There is controversy over the association between undermining and pressure ulcer infection. (Undermining refers to the extension of the lesion under the skin such that the wound cavity is larger than the surface opening.) Bliss (1993) has stated that undermining is not related to infection but is caused by proteolytic lysis of dermal tissues. However, Bliss did not consider that the proteases may be of bacterial origin. Conversely, Sibbald *et al* (2003) argues that undermining may be the result of bacterial digestion or prevention of granulation tissue formation. Some bacteria produce proteolytic enzymes known as invasins (Cooper, 2003) that digest protein and extracellular matrix components, so enlarging the wound.

The criterion of pain requires careful consideration with respect to infection. Damage or irritation to peripheral nerves (neuropathic pain) may be a component of pressure ulcer development (Reddy *et al*, 2003). If infection intervenes the pain is likely to increase and erythema and induration, more than 2cm from the wound edge, may well be concurrent manifestations (Reddy *et al*, 2003) (*Table 7.4*) (*Figure 7.3*).

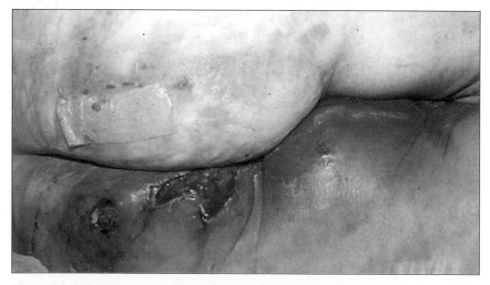

Figure 7.3: Infected pressure ulcer of the buttocks, with cellulitis

Acute and surgical wounds

Many clinicians rely on the classical signs of infection (pain, erythema, oedema, heat and purulence) to identify infection in this type of wound. Although these are often relevant, the infection detection rate is dependent on the criteria used. This fact is clearly demonstrated by Ayliffe *et al* (1977) who showed that a wound infection prevalence rate of 15.6% (of a sample of 3354 wounds) dropped to 6.9% when pus was the only criterion for infection. Suggested criteria for acute or surgical wound infection are listed in *Table 7.5* with provision made for wounds that are healing through either primary or secondary intention (*Figure 7.4*).

Table 7.4: Signs of infection of pressure ulcers

- Erythema[5]
- Oedema[5]
- Pain/tenderness — change in nature of pain[5]
- Discolouration[6]
- Increase in exudate volume[6]
- Delayed healing[6]

(NB when multiple sclerosis is present pain is not a criterion)

5. National Pressure Ulcer Advisory Panel (2000) Frequently asked questions, wound infection and infection control. Online at: http://www.npuap.org/woundinfection.htm (accessed 20 February 2004)

6. Cutting KF, Harding KG (1994) Criteria for identifing wound infection. *J Wound Care* 3(4): 198–201

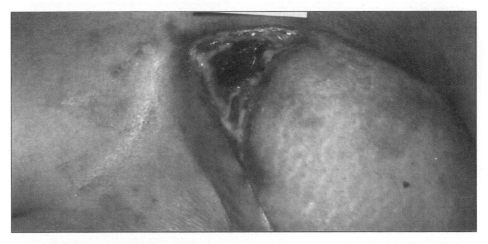

Figure 7.4: Infected surgical wound

Venous leg ulcers

The presence of lipodermatosclerosis and haemosiderin staining can mask features such as erythema, and pain is a common characteristic of these ulcers even without infection. Therefore, the permutation of signs and symptoms must be interpreted in context of patient familiarity, notably changes in presentation (*Table 7.6*) (*Figure 7.5*).

Table 7.5: Signs of infection of acute/surgical wounds

Primary closed wounds

- Abscess[6]
- Cellulitis[6]
- Discharge (serous exudate with inflammation, seropurulent, haemopurulent, pus)[6]
- Delayed healing[6]
- Discolouration[6]
- Unexpected pain/tenderness[6]
- Bridging of the epithelium or soft tissue[6]
- Abnormal smell[6]
- Wound breakdown[6]

Wound healing by secondary intention

- Abscess/pus[7]
- Heat[7]
- Oedema[7]
- Erythema[7]
- Cellulitis[6]
- Discharge (serous exudate with inflammation, seropurulent, haemopurulent, pus)[7]
- Delayed healing[7]
- Discolouration[7]
- Friable granulation tissue which bleeds easily[7]
- Unexpected pain/tenderness[7]
- Bridging of the epithelium or soft tissue[6]
- Pocketing at the base of wound[8]
- Abnormal smell[7]
- Wound breakdown

6. Cutting KF, Harding KG (1994) Criteria for identifying wound infection. *J Wound Care* **3**(4): 198–201
7. Gardner SE, Frantz RA, Doebbeling BN (2001) The validity of the clinical signs and symptoms used to identify localized chronic wound infection. *Wound Repair Regen* **9**(3): 78–186
8. Marks J, Harding KG, Hughes LE, Ribeiro CD (1985) Pilondial sinus excision — healing by open granulation. *Br J Surg* **72**: 637–40

Arterial leg ulcers

Arterial ulcers of purely ischaemic aetiology exist independently of cutaneous haemosiderin deposits (as is the case with venous and complex ulcers). Consequently, the skin is ostensibly normal in appearance with erythema clearly evident (*Figure 7.6*). As with ischaemic diabetic foot ulcers, the redness of erythema may be difficult to distinguish from the erythema of cellulitis. Furthermore, infection (*Table 7.7*) may present as bluish-purple discolouration of soft tissues, owing to the increased metabolic demands of infection, combined with reduced blood flow to the skin secondary to septic vasculitis of the cutaneous circulation (Edmonds and Foster, 2000).

Full-thickness burns

Third degree burns (*Table 7.8*), particularly after tangential excision, are generally anaesthetic therefore pain is not always an infection criterion. Similarly, erythema as a result of infection may not be distinct from normal wound inflammation. Increase in the level of exudate from infection is also difficult or impossible to determine because of the high volume of fluid produced in full-thickness burns.

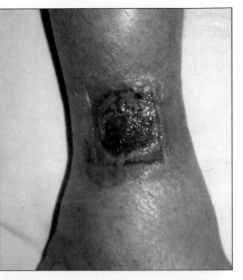

Figure 7.5: Venous leg ulcer infected by *Pseudomonas aeruginosa*

Table 7.6: Signs of infection of venous leg ulcers

- Discolouration
- Dull brick red (ß-haemolytic *streptococci*)[9]
- Blue/green (*Pseudomonas aeruginosa*)[6]
- Delayed healing[7]
- Increased serous exudateÈ[6]
- Cellulitis[6]
- Change in the nature of pain[7]

NB: lipodermatosclerosis and haemosiderin staining of the skin can confuse palpable and some visual signs of infection

6. Cutting KF, Harding KG (1994) Criteria for identifying wound infection. *J Wound Care* **3**(4): 198–201
7. Gardner SE, Frantz RA, Doebbeling BN (2001) The validity of the clinical signs and symptoms used to identify localized chronic wound infection. *Wound Repair Regen* **9**(3): 78–186
9. Schraibman IG (1990) The significance of beta-haemolytic streptococci in chronic leg ulcers. *Ann R Coll Surg Engl* **72**(2): 123–4

Discussion

The development of the above criteria may be considered as an interim measure as they reflect current observation and understanding. The next step is to review the development of wound infection criteria in light of current knowledge. In 1994 Cutting and Harding's understanding of infection did not include the concept of critical colonization, a stage in the infection continuum (Sibbald *et al*, 2000; Kingsley, 2001). Critical colonization has traditionally been perceived as a theoretical concept, but it is now gaining acceptance. The wound infection continuum (Kingsley, 2001; White, 2003) is a concept that illustrates the possible transition of a wound from sterility to infection (*Figure 7.7*). Research-based publications (eg. Fumal *et al*, 2002; Wall *et al*, 2002 and Stephens *et al*, 2003) and a review (Edwards and Harding, 2004) have served to confirm critical colonization as a reality rather than a concept.

At the point of critical colonization the wound has become compromised (Cutting, 2003). Current thinking would support the notion that, at this stage, the wound is not demonstrating any visible clues to this compromised situation.

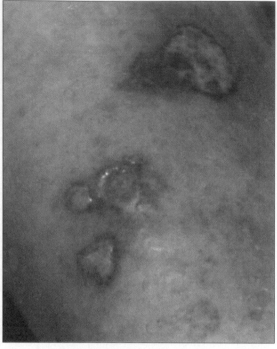

Figure 7.6: Infected arterial leg ulcers

But is this correct? Is the wound on the brink of infection and only demonstrating this with indolence or recalcitrance or are clues present that we have not yet identified? Critical colonization implies the inability to maintain a balance between the increasing numbers of bacteria and an effective immune system. Perhaps this circumstance is influencing the situation in ways that we do not yet understand. The need therefore exists to investigate, develop and subsequently validate clinical signs of infection that will assist in identifying not only infection but also critical colonization. It should be remembered that the identification of infection is dependent on the criteria used, a notion which is supported by Wilson *et al* (1990). Detection is clearly the impetus for treatment and therefore will have a major impact on morbidity.

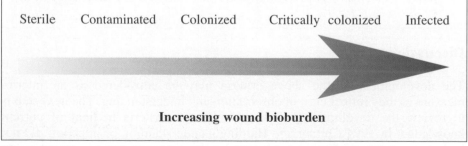

Figure 7.7: The original wound infection continuum (subsequently modified)

If the wound progresses to the final stage in the infection continuum, the clinical signs become 'more obvious' although some may remain subtle in nature (eg. *Figure 7.8*). The above collation of criteria according to wound type has been prepared for a number of reasons. Firstly, to raise awareness that criteria for infection may vary with wound type. Secondly, application of these criteria provides the potential for early detection of wound infection. Thirdly, to encourage reflection on individual use of clinical criteria, stimulting debate and ultimately generating consensus.

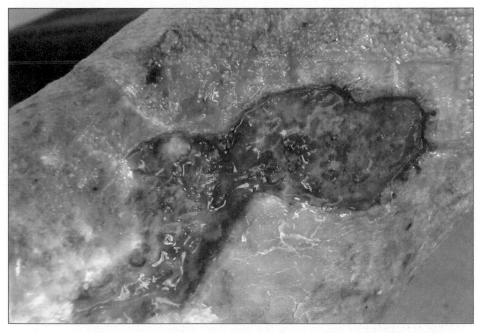

Figure 7.8: Venous leg ulcer infected with *Pseudomonas aeruginosa* and ß-haemolytic *streptococci*, but displaying only subtle signs of infection — the upper two-thirds of the wound is darker than the rest

Table 7.7: Signs of infection of arterial leg ulcers
• Erythema or bluish-purple peri-ulcer soft tissues[10]
• Pain[10]
• Increased exudate[10]
• Malodour[10]
• Palpable crepitus from gas in soft tissues[11]
• Heat[10]
• Turgor[10]

10. Edmonds M, Foster AVM (2000) *Managing the Diabetc Foot*. Blackwell Science Ltd, Oxford
11. Sapico F, Bessman A (1991) Diabetic foot infections. In: Fryberg R, ed. *The High Risk Foot in Diabetes Mellitus*. Churchill Livingstone, New York

Table 7.8: Signs of infection of full thickness burns

- Graft rejection[12]

12. Krupp S, Baechler M, Bille J (1985) Assessment of burn wound sepsis. *J Hosp Infect* **6**(Suppl A): 133–7

Conclusion

Although the 1994 wound infection criteria remain a useful tool in the identification of wound infection, they currently offer a 'catch all' approach. It is considered that the development of criteria specific to six different wound types is essential if improvements or advancements are to made in the identification of wound infection, in order to decrease the time spent between the onset of infection and its effective treatment, and to decrease patient morbidity. Whether the early detection of critical colonization is feasible remains to be seen.

Key points

⌘ The current standard criteria for wound infection are generic, based on empirical data, and now ten years old.

⌘ There is ample justification for revisiting these criteria on a wound type basis.

⌘ This exercise has been conducted using a Delphi expert panel approach.

⌘ Preliminary findings for six wound types are reported.

⌘ Practitioners are urged to use these criteria in their clinical practice in order to reduce patient morbidity, and, spare antibiotic use.

References

Armstrong DG, Lavery LA, Saraya M, Ashry H (1996) Leukocytosis is a poor indicator of acute osteomyelitis of the foot in diabetes mellitus. *J Foot Ankle Surgery* **35**(4): 280–3

Ayliffe GAJ, Brightwell KM, Collins BJ *et al* (1977) Surveys of hospital infection in the Birmingham region. *J Hygiene* (London) **79**: 299–314

Bliss M (1993) Aetiology of pressure sores. *Reviews in Clinical Gerontology* **3**: 379–97

Boulton AJM, Bowker JH (1985) The diabetic foot. In: Olefsky JM, Serwin R, eds. *Diabetes Mellitus: Management and Complications*. Churchill Livingstone, New York

Bowler PG, Davies BJ, Jones SA (1999) Microbial involvement in chronic wound malodour. *J Wound Care* **8**(5): 216–18

Cooper RA (2003) The contribution of microbial virulence to wound infection. In: White RJ, ed. *The Silver Book*. Quay Books, MA Healthcare Limited, Dinton, Salisbury, Wiltshire

Cutting KF (1998) The identification of infection in granulating wounds by registered nurses. *J Clin Nurs* **7**(6): 539–46

Cutting KF (2003) Wound healing, bacteria and topical therapies. *EWMA Journal* **3**(1): 17–19

Cutting KF, Harding KG (1994) Criteria for identifying wound infection. *J Wound Care* **3**(4): 198–201

Edmonds ME, Foster AVM (2000) *Managing the Diabetic Foot*. Blackwell Science Ltd, Oxford

Edwards R, Harding KG (2004) Bacteria and wound healing. *Current Opinion Infect Dis* **17**(2): 91–6

Fumal I, Braham C, Paquet P, Pierard-Franchimont C, Pierard GE (2002) The beneficial toxicity paradox of antimicrobials in leg ulcer healing impaired by a polymicrobial flora: A proof-of-concept study. *Dermatology* **204**(Suppl 1):70–4

Gardner SE, Frantz RA, Doebbeling BN (2001) The validity of the clinical signs and symptoms used to identify localized chronic wound infection. *Wound Repair Regen* **9**(3): 78–186

Heggers JP 1998. Defining infection in chronic wounds: does it matter? *J Wound Care* **7**(8):389-392.

Jones J, Hunter D (1995) Consensus methods for medical and health services research. *Br Med J* **311**(7001): 376–80

Kingsley A (2001) A proactive approach to wound infection. *Nurs Stand* **15**(30): 50–8

Leaper DJ (1998) Defining infection: Editorial. *J Wound Care* **7**(8): 373

Marks J, Harding KG, Hughes LE, Ribeiro CD (1985) Pilonidal sinus excision – healing by open granulation. *Br J Surgery* **72**: 637–40

Reddy M, Keast D, Fowler E, Sibbald GS (2003) Pain in pressure ulcers. *Ostomy Wound Manage* **49**(4 Suppl): 30–5

Serralta VW, Harrison-Balestra C, Cazzaniga AL, Davis SC, Mertz PM (2001). Lifestyles of bacteria in wounds: presence of biofilms? *Wounds* **13**(1): 29–34

Sibbald RG, Williamson D, Orsted HL et al (2000) Preparing the wound bed: debridement, bacterial balance and moisture balance. *Ostomy Wound Manage* **46**(11): 14–35

Sibbald RG, Orsted H, Schultz GS, Coutts P, Keast D (2003) Preparing the wound bed 2003: Focus on infection and inflammation. *Ostomy Wound Manage* **49**(11): 24–51

Stephens, P, Wall IB, Wilson MJ (2003) Cutaneous biology: anaerobic cocci populating the deep tissues of chronic wounds impair cellular wound healing responses in vitro. *Br J Dermatol* **148**: 456–66

Wall IB, Davies CE, Hill KE et al (2002) Potential role of anaerobic cocci in impaired human wound healing. *Wound Repair Regen* **10**(6): 346–53

White RJ (2003) The wound infection continuum. In: White RJ, ed. *Trends in Wound Care, volume II*. Quay Books, MA Healthcare Limited, Dinton, Salisbury: 12–18

Wilson AP, Weavill C, Burridge J, Kelsey MC, (1990) The use of the wound scoring method 'ASEPSIS' in postoperative wound surveillance. *J Hosp Infect* **16**(4): 297–309

8

Health-related quality of life tools for venous-ulcerated patients

SC Anand, C Dean, R Nettleton, DV Praburaj

Healthcare manufacturing companies have developed many new and novel materials for wound care. They claim that the dressing materials will improve the healing progress of the wound or have a therapeutic value and have sought to assess their efficacy and effectiveness in clinical trials. These claims should be clearly supported by the perspectives of those who actually use the devices. Compression therapy, which is regarded as an effective treatment for venous leg ulcers, is far from ideal owing to a number of limitations that it possesses, such as patient discomfort, difficulty experienced in applying correct compression on the limbs, choosing a correct dressing for the wound or finding differences between the performance of various devices. It is necessary to investigate the patient's views and perspectives while randomized controlled clinical trials are conducted. In this review the concept of quality of life (QoL) and the tools used to measure QoL and studies that were conducted with patients suffering from chronic venous leg ulcers and undergoing therapy are considered, along with contributory factors to the healing process. In addition, a questionnaire modified from the original format is recommended as the suitable tool for assessing the QoL of patients suffering from venous leg ulcers while participating in clinical trials.

An ideal clinical trial in wound care would be a well-planned prospective study conducted on patients comparing the effects of devices by a process of randomization, so that a clearly formed question can be answered (Venkatraman *et al*, 2002a, b). Most clinical trials evaluating the efficacy of wound care dressing modalities rely only on objective medical assessments such as mean healing time of wound, closure of wound, and absorption of exudate, and ignore the subjective perspectives of patients like quality of life (QoL).

In chronic venous leg-ulcerated patients, elimination or cure of disease (ie. patient reverting to ambulation and restoring to normal healthy lifestyle) is not attainable and the treatment could be longer than first anticipated. A plethora of wound dressings and bandages are used to assist the treatment of venous ulcers, and have an impact on patients' wellbeing. A study conducted by Callam *et al* (1987) found that venous leg ulcers affect greatly the life of patients and their mobility, causing people a significant burden to life. Hence, assessing QoL while administering new dressing products to patients, in addition to the objective evaluations, is likely to be an essential assessment while gathering evidence on medical devices in clinical trials.

The main aims of this review are to: explore the concept of QoL; evaluate the measurement tools used to assess an individual's views or perspectives on treatment; review the studies conducted in this area; and identify a relevant questionnaire from the published literature to assess the perspectives of patients suffering from venous leg ulcers while participating in clinical trials evaluating the performance of medical devices.

An extensive search was carried out in the journals: *Journal of Wound Care* (1993–2000), *Journal of Wound, Ostomy and Continence Nursing* (1996–2001), *Phlebology* (1992–2001), and online databases: Ovid Bibliographic Records, Medline (1993 to present) for the key words venous leg ulcers, quality of life tools, compression therapy and trials evaluating QoL as an outcome measure to find out those studies evaluating treatment and assessing QoL.

Venous leg ulcer

A venous leg ulcer is an irregular-shaped deep- or partial-thickness wound with well defined borders, generally surrounded by hyperpigmented indurated skin. A yellow-white exudate may be seen. These ulcers vary in size and location, but they are usually found in the gaiter area. Oedema is common in the ankle region. Tissue infection can also occur. Pain is reported while in motion, during standing and while at rest (Zimmet, 1999). The calf muscle pump initiates the return of blood from the lower limb back to the heart. The calf pump mechanism consists of calf muscles, the deep venous system and the superficial venous compartment connected to deep veins through one-way valves via perforator veins. Malfunctioning of any of these components can lead to venous ulceration (Zimmet, 1999).

Compression therapy is considered to be an effective non-operative treatment for patients with uninfected or infected venous ulcers (Zimmet, 1999; Moneta *et al*, 2000). Compression is achieved by producing a pressure gradient highest at the ankle and gradually reducing towards the calf region just below the knee (Zimmet, 1999). Wound dressings which are used include foams and alginates for significant amount of wound exudate, hydrocolloids and hydrogel for mild to moderate drainage, and films for superficial wounds. These wound dressings maintain a moist environment that accelerates autolytic debridement of dead tissue, reduces pain and facilitates simpler wound care (Zimmet, 1999).

The problem of venous ulceration in UK

Venous ulceration affects nearly 1–2% of the UK population (80,000–100,000 patients at any one time), and a further 400,000 patients experience recurrence (Morison *et al*, 1998). Occurrence increases as age increases from 10 per 1000 within adult population (less than sixty-five years) to 36 per 1,000 in the age range of sixty-five and above, and is predominant in women (Bale *et al*, 1997). Also, there are reports that a minor proportion of people below the age of 40 years suffer from venous leg ulcers (Bennett and Moody, 1995; Morison *et al*, 1998).

Leg ulcer management costs £600 million per year, and approximately 2% of the budget of the NHS resources is spent on the management of venous diseases (Marlow, 1999). A conservative estimate of £1200 is spent on every patient per annum based on a visit per week by a district nurse. Factors influencing the cost of treatment include time to heal, use of dressing regime, and ability to prevent recurrence and QoL (Nelzén, 2000).

Benefits of compression therapy

The primary function of elastic compression therapy is to control the oedema or swelling of tissues and to aid the return of venous blood from the lower limb to the heart. This is supported by appropriate primary contact dressings, such as moisture-retentive dressings and absorbent dressings, to create a moist environment to progress healing of the wound (Thomas, 2001).

Compression therapy is the favourable alternative to other forms of compression systems (pneumatic compression devices, electrical stimulation, hyperbaric oxygen, ultrasound and low-intensity laser therapy [Zimmet, 1999]), in returning the venous blood back to the heart by applying recommended external pressure to the lower limbs via compression bandages (Moneta *et al*, 2000). Elastic compression stockings, Unna's boot and multilayer compression bandages are claimed to achieve excellent healing rates (Moneta *et al*, 2000). In a review by Mayberry *et al* (1991), 113 patients were managed with compression therapy over fifteen years, of which 102 patients were compliant. The authors report that 75% of ulcers can be healed in six months' time and up to 90% can be successfully treated within one year of using elastic compression systems in the compliant patients.

Limitations of compression therapy

Although compression is a cornerstone for treating venous-ulcerated patients, health professionals claim that there are many limitations to its use, such as discomfort and intolerance, resulting in poor compliance. Elastic stockings have been reported to be not tolerated initially in hypersensitive areas adjacent to an active wound or in a previously healed ulcer. High pressures applied initially to the wound also contribute to intolerance. Ambulant patients find it difficult to reach their feet in order to put the stockings on, or find it uncomfortable while wearing shoes (Moneta *et al*, 2000).

Unna's boot, a paste bandage widely used in the USA (Moneta *et al*, 2000), has many limitations: the application of the dressings is labour intensive and expensive; achieving the right degree of compression is dependent on the carer's or nurse's experience; it is uncomfortable to wear as it becomes rigid once it is dry; and it has been reported to cause inflammation of the skin because of the preservative added in the mixture (Moneta *et al*, 2000). Moreover, the bandage needs replacing when excess drainage is observed in the limb as it is not designed to absorb exudate, and the physician cannot monitor the wound healing progress once the boot is applied.

Multilayer compression bandages are reported to achieve a better healing rate with painless healing (Moneta *et al*, 2000). Although this bandage achieves sustained pressure it is reported to be uncomfortable, and achieving the correct compression is nurse-dependent.

Elastic stockings are knitted with elastic fibres capable of recovering their size and shape after deformation. According to Veraat *et al* (1997a), the pressure applied by the stocking was 18.3mmHg (or 74% below the required amount). These stockings did not provide the adequate compression which is required to improve ulcer healing in the medial side of the leg. When washed and used repeatedly, there is a deterioration in compression pressure in elastic stockings (Veraat *et al*, 1997b).

It is necessary to study the limitations of compression therapy modalities, tolerance, compliance and comfort by investigating the patient's perspectives on bandages and dressings when they are evaluated for efficacy in clinical trials.

Health-related quality of life (HRQoL)

Quality of life is a broad term; it means different things to different people and it takes many forms depending on the specific circumstances and conditions under which the term is applied. The World Health Organization (WHO) has defined health as a state of complete physical, mental and social wellbeing and not merely absence of disease (WHO, 1976, 1984).

Quality of life is a subjective assessment of patients' welfare and is influenced by various factors beyond the health status (Nettleton, 2002, unpublished observations). However, in the context of clinical trials evaluating medical devices on patients, researchers interpret this broader term as the impact of disease on the normal functioning of patients in addition to the effect of treatment on the patient's health (Fayers and Machin, 2000). This can also be referred to as health-related quality of life.

Many experts in this field report that QoL is a multidimensional construct that covers issues relating to general health, physical functioning, physical symptoms, toxic effects, sleep, emotional functioning, social, sexual and occupational functioning (Price, 1993; Reid, 1996; Fayers and Machin, 2000). Price (1993) defines QoL as a wider concept that reflects the individual's perspectives on the level of satisfaction experienced in a variety of circumstances. Price (1993) emphasizes people's views on their happiness relative to their life in general.

Quality of life is generally measured by asking patients to answer a set of closed questions. These questions, which can be single or multi-items, are used to assess the perspectives of patients. There are two types of HRQoL-tools, namely generic tools and disease-specific tools (*Table 8.1*). Generic tools cover a wide range of dimensions and are used with a variety of diseases (*Table 8.2*). Some examples include the Nottingham health profile (NHP) (Hunt *et al*, 1985) and the short form-36 (SF-36) (Ware and Sherbourne, 1992). These tools are designed to measure the impact of disease or disorder on the daily functioning of patients (Price, 1998). Disease-specific tools cover measures that are directly related to a particular disease, hence they have better sensitivity to detect the minor changes or symptoms observed in patients suffering from a particular illness (Price, 1993).

The reasons why QoL should be incorporated as an outcome in studies evaluating the effectiveness of treatment for venous leg ulcers include the factors listed in *Table 8.3*.

Table 8.1: Type of quality of life questionnaires

Generic tool: Nottingham health profile (NHP) (Hunt *et al*, 1985); Short-form health survey (SF-36) (Ware and Sherbourne, 1992); McGill pain questionnaire (SF-MPQ) (Melzack, 1975); Frenchay activities index (FAI) (Holbrock and Skilbeck, 1983); EuroQol (EQ) (de Charro, 2001)

Disease-specific tool: Cardiff wound impact schedule (CWIS) (Price and Harding, 1997); Hyland new ulcer specific tool (Hyland and Thompson, 1994); Charing Cross venous leg ulcer questionnaire (Smith *et al*, 2000); Freiburger questionnaire (FLQA) (Augustin *et al*, 1997); Chronic venous insufficiency questionnaire (CIVIQ) (Launois *et al*, 1996)

Table 8.2: Advantages and disadvantages of generic tools

Advantages: The questionnaire is general in format; the measuring tool is validated; the tool can be used with confidence; the tool can be used to compare various diseases; the results of the study can be compared across groups of patients with different health characteristics (Price, 1993)

Disadvantages: The items are broad; the questions may be irrelevant or vague for particular disease patients; single scores can be insensitive to changes over time (Price, 1993), ie. failure to detect the variations observed on patients over a period

Table 8.3: Reasons why quality of life (QoL) should be incorporated as an outcome in studies

QoL can be used in those clinical trials which are evaluating the therapy or treatment or medical devices and can assess the benefit of one treatment or device to the other. When comparing two treatment or devices, QoL tools can be used to assess the benefits that one treatment possesses over the other

To investigate the advantages and disadvantages of new medical devices

In some diseases complete cure is unattainable or may be a long-term process, hence assessing QoL is likely to be an essential measure

Success or failure of a treatment can be determined by assessing the QoL

When the efficacy of two devices evaluated in a clinical trial are found to be equivalent, the device associated with a better QoL score is more likely to be adopted for clinical practice (Marlow, 1999)

Short-term efficacy of specific treatments may differ considerably, but if the overall failure rate of the treatment modality is high then QoL can be considered as a significant measure (Fayers and Machin, 2000)

QoL can be a main end point in clinical trials evaluating treatment devices on chronic incurable diseases

Health professionals making decisions about cost-effective treatment methods consider QoL as an important measure (Marlow, 1999)

Literature review

The following section reviews studies that were conducted on this subject and are summarized in *Table 8.4*.

Lindholm *et al* (1993) reported the use of the short version of Nottingham health profile (NHP) on 125 patients (seventy-four females and fifty-one males) who were suffering from venous ulcers for more than six months. They report that men had generally higher scores than women in all the QoL areas (a high score indicates poor QoL).

Franks and Moffat (1998) reported the use of NHP on 758 leg ulcer patients in six community trusts. This cross-sectional study compared the scores of NHP with the age/sex matched with the normal scores (normal scores are the standard scores obtained from healthy participants studied nationwide) obtained from a previous published study result using NHP by Hunt *et al* (1984) that used the above questionnaire on patients. All the participants reported poor HRQoL in all domains of the questionnaire (energy, pain, emotional reactions, sleep, social isolation and physical mobility).

Comparing NHP scores with sex-matched normal scores between men and women, the authors found that women experienced less energy, disturbed sleep patterns, lack of mobility, emotional reactions, increased physical pain and social isolation compared with men. The authors also add that the mean differences were greater for the younger age group (age less than sixty-five years) than the older patients (sixty-five years and above). Thus, younger patients experienced poorer QoL and men scored higher than women in the domains of body pain, sleep and social isolation.

Health-related quality of life was assessed using the NHP in a recent prospective randomized parallel group trial of two bandage systems by Franks *et al* (1999). The original four-layer system (ninety-nine patients) was compared with the Profore (Smith & Nephew) four-layer compression bandage system (109 patients). The patients were asked to complete the survey at the start, at twelve weeks and at twenty-four weeks. The authors report that at twenty-four weeks, 167 patients whose ulcers had healed noticed significant improvements in sleep, bodily pain and mobility as opposed to forty-one patients whose ulcers remained unhealed. In the rest of the domains there were no significant differences between the original and the Profore group of patients.

Price and Harding (1996) conducted a study to identify the usefulness of the short-form survey (SF-36) questionnaire to measure the quality of life of sixty-three patients suffering from venous leg ulcers who attended a specialist wound-healing clinic. The results from the study suggest that when describing the functional status and wellbeing of the patients, the SF-36 questionnaire served the purpose. The data from the study were compared with UK norms data obtained previously on healthy controls in age range seventy to seventy-four years (Jenkinson *et al*, 1993).

The eight subscales of SF-36 were scored on a scale from 0 as worst possible health state and 100 as best possible health state. The results showed that seven out of eight subscales were significantly different, such that patients were experiencing more pain, less energy, more restriction in physical and social functioning, and poorer health and limitations in physical and emotional roles. However, the authors stress the need for a disease-specific questionnaire to further the research by comparing the SF-36 with a condition-specific tool.

Walters *et al* (1999) compared four generic tools — SF-36, Euroqol (EQ), short-form McGill pain (SF-MPQ), and Frenchay activities index (FAI). This study took into account the two main properties, namely discriminative property and evaluative property, which are the requirements of a HRQoL tool. The study was conducted on 233 venous ulcer patients as part of a randomized clinical trial evaluating the cost-effectiveness of community leg ulcer clinics. They evaluated two important requirements of a HRQoL tool; namely, discriminative properties (capacity to differentiate patients with or without ulcers at a point of time) and evaluative properties (capacity to measure the change in HRQoL within a patient over time in response to a treatment).

The authors report that during the initial assessment, SF-MPQ had a poor ability to distinguish different patient groups than the other three tools (SF-36, FAI and EQ) in relation to age and ulcer duration. Frenchay activities index had the ability to differentiate different patient groups in relation to age, mobility and ulcer size during initial assessment. The SF-36 contained items that questions patients' health status at present and within the past four weeks; FAI asks about frequency of activities from three to six months; EQ asks about health status on the day of completion, eg. when comparing the health status over time from baseline (start) to three-month follow-up, EQ questions patients' HRQoL only on the day of completion of the study. The SF-MPQ asks patients questions on their health status at present time and the pain experienced by patients in the past week. In FAI, the questions refer to HRQoL from three to six months, hence it cannot detect the changes in health of patients in a three-month trial.

The authors recommend SF-MPQ for short-term follow-up (three-month), as it had good property to measure changes in health of patient associated to ulcer healing over time. For a long-term period (twelve months) SF-36 and EQ showed good evaluative properties. However, FAI was not sensitive to detect the differences in HRQoL over time between patients whose ulcer was healed or not. SF-MPQ was the only instrument that detected the difference between the groups of patients whose ulcer healed or not, in small sample size. Hence, Walters *et al* (1999) recommend SF-MPQ during the evaluation of devices with short-term follow-up (three months) and the SF-36 tool during the long-term follow-up.

Smith *et al* (2000) validated a newly designed disease-specific questionnaire called the Charing Cross venous leg ulcer questionnaire. The study was conducted on ninety-eight venous leg ulcer patients (fifty-eight women and forty men), who completed both the SF-36 questionnaire and the new tool. The new tool was assessed for its validity, reliability and responsiveness. The new ulcer-specific questionnaire showed a highly significant negative correlation (correlations significant at 1% level) in all the eight domains of SF-36. The correlations were negative because the ulcer-specific tool measured 100 as the worst possible situation, while SF-36 measured 100 as the best possible health. The correlations exceeded 0.5 in absolute magnitude for all the domains.

Table 8.4: List of questionnaires and their outcomes (to be continued)

Name of the instrument (acronym)	Author of the tool	Issues covered (items)	Application	Studies conducted using the tool
Nottingham health profile (NHP)	Hunt *et al* (1985)	38-item instrument that covers various domains: physical mobility (8), pain (8), social isolation (5), emotional reactions (9), energy (3) and sleep (5)	Extensively reported in asthma and is used for evaluating perceived distress across various populations, well validated and widely used in clinical research	Three different studies were conducted: Lindholm *et al* (1993), Franks and Moffat (1998), and Franks *et al* (1999)
Short-form health survey (SF-36)	Ware and Sherbourne (1992)	36 items are covered: physical functioning (10), social functioning (2), energy (4), body pain (2), mental health (5), physical role limitation (4), emotional problems (3) and general health (6)	Originated in the USA and is used in elderly patients suffering from various diseases	Price and Harding, (1996) assessed the usefulness of the SF-36 and compared with normative data on 63 patients suffering from venous ulcers
Short-form McGill pain questionnaire (SF MPQ)	Melzack (1975)	The shorter version consists of 15 questions or pain descriptors rated on intensity scale suffering from venous leg ulcers	Designed to generate a quantitative measure of pain used in all type of diseases	Walters *et al* (1999) compared and contrasted four generic questionnaires on patients
Frenchay activities index (FAI)	Holbrock and Skilbeck (1983)	Day-to-day activities are recorded over the past 3 months. Domestic chores, leisure or work and outdoor activities	Designed for patients with stroke, intended to measure activities of level of independence in older people	Walters *et al* (1999) compared and contrasted four generic questionnaires on patients
EuroQol (EQ)	de Charro (2001)	One-page tool consists of five questions on mobility, self-care, usual activities, pain and anxiety/depression	Used on wide range of health conditions and is designed to complement the, SF-36 NHP and other disease-specific tools	A comparison of four different generic questionnaires on patients by Walters *et al* (1999)
Hyland new ulcer specific tool	Hyland and Thompson (1994)	Functional limitations and emotional reactions of patients	A new tool for patients suffering from chronic wounds	Hyland and Thompson (1994) outlined the development of the new tool
Cardiff wound impact schedule (CWIS)	Price and Harding (1997)	Tool is divided into four sections: physical symptoms and daily living (12), social (7), wellbeing (7) and overall HRQol (2)	A condition-specific tool used to assess quality of life of patients suffering from chronic venous wounds	Price and Harding (2000) reported the use of tool on acute and chronic wounds
Charing cross venous leg ulcer questionnaire	Smith *et al* (2000)	Psychometric properties: social function, domestic activities, cosmesis and emotional status (22 items)	Ulcer-specific questionnaire validated against the SF-36	Smith *et al* (2000) demonstrated the validity and reliability of the questionnaire

Table 8.4 (continued): List of questionnaires and their outcomes				
Name of the instrument (acronym)	Author of the tool	Issues covered (items)	Application	Studies conducted using the tool
Freiburger Lebensqualitäts assessment questionnaire (FLQA)	Augustin et al (1997)	Consists of 83 items: physical complaints, everyday life, social life, emotional status, therapy, satisfaction, and occupation	A German language questionnaire designed to examine health measures in chronic venous disease	Augustin et al reported the 1997 results of the pilot study conducted on 246 patients validating the questionnaire
Chronic venous insufficiency questionnaire (CVIQ)	Launois et al (1996)	Psychosocial, physical functioning, social functioning and pain	A 20-item questionnaire designed specifically to reflect the perspectives of patients suffering from venous insufficiency	Vayssairat et al (2000) reported the use of CIVIQ in a 4-week efficacy trial

Smith *et al* (2000) claim that high correlation of venous ulcer-specific questionnaire scores with all eight domains of SF-36 was because the ulcer questionnaire was picking up the adverse effects of venous ulceration. The patients were asked to fill the questionnaire at six and twelve weeks. The responsiveness of the tool was shown by a significant reduction in the scores of ulcer questionnaire whose venous ulcers had healed. However, the tool is yet to show its effectiveness in clinical trials evaluating treatment devices.

Price and Harding (1997) used a new tool, the Cardiff wound impact schedule (CWIS), to investigate the factors which patients find stressful when experiencing chronic ulcers at two points in time by asking them to rate items from a checklist. The authors report the impact of the wound on the patient's QoL and they add that ratings obtained at the first time were different from the second time, as the response from patients tends to change over time. Price and Harding (2000) reported the use of CWIS tool in acute wounds (seventeen patients) and chronic wounds (thirty-two patients) treated in a specialist clinic. The study outcome revealed that chronic ulceration had a greater impact on physical and social functioning and wellbeing of patients. However, when rating the overall HRQoL, patients with chronic wounds rated better. The authors conclude that the QoL deteriorates with increasing age where chronic ulceration is more prevalent.

Hyland and Thompson (1994) described the process of development of a new ulcer-specific tool from initial interviews, focus groups and a pilot study. The fifty-four-item tool consists of three sections: section one covers patients' details and whether the ulcer is getting better or worse; section two covers items related to the level of pain, sleep disturbance, time spent on the ulcer and thinking about the ulcer; and section three discusses functional limitations, dysphoric mood and treatment.

The study demonstrated that patients were facing problems owing to pain, disturbance of sleep and restricted movement. However, there were no reports of use of the tool in randomized controlled trials (RCTs). In addition, the authors report that the sample size (*n*=50) used for this analysis is insufficient and that further research is needed in using the tool.

Chronic venous insufficiency questionnaire (CIVIQ) is a twenty-item disease-specific questionnaire developed by Launois *et al* (1996) for patients suffering from lower limb venous insufficiency. The authors report the development of the tool from a pilot study of twenty patients, identifying critical features that affect the venous leg ulcer patients, to a larger study of 2001 patients that aided them to reduce the number of items. The questionnaire was tested on sixty patients at first and then tested again on the same set of subjects to find its reproducibility. The questionnaire was also tested in a large-scale RCT consisting of 934 patients, thus evaluating the patient response and validity of the tool.

The results from the trial found that the questionnaire may be used with confidence on chronic venous insufficiency in clinical trials. Vayssairat *et al* (2000) also reported the use of this tool in a four-week efficacy trial comparing class I elastic compression stockings (10–15mmHg) with placebo stockings (3–6mmHg). The symptoms index that represents the sum of individual scores for pain, limb heaviness, cramps, paresthesias and evening limb oedema were assessed. Statistically significant differences (*P*=0.05) were obtained in the QoL in favour of class I elastic compression stocking.

Augustin *et al* (1997) developed the Freiburger Lebensqualitäts assessment questionnaire (FLQA). The development of the tool started with open questions used to identify those factors that would affect patients. The eighty-three-item questionnaire obtained was piloted to test the acceptance and consistency of the tool. The authors studied the outcome of the tool on 246 patients with chronic venous insufficiency in a university clinic and compared the longitudinal study results with NHP and Questionnaire Alltagsleben scores (ALLTAG) (Bullinger *et al*, 1993). The authors claim the instrument to be valid by obtaining high correlations with NHP and ALLTAG. Reliability was also high and the feasibility of the tool was satisfactory since the rate of missing data was less than 5%. However, patients with severe illness and elderly debilitating patients were not included in their study and only people with good command of German can use the tool.

Specific measurements in the QoL tool relation to venous leg ulcers

Several disease-specific measurement tools have been developed in order to reflect the patients' views of their health specific to a particular disease, namely venous leg ulcer. Several generic questionnaires were compared and contrasted by Walters *et al* (1999) and they recommend use of SF-MPQ while evaluating devices with short-term follow-up (three months), and the SF-36 tool during the long-term follow-up. Different closed-end ulcer-specific questionnaires have been developed because generic questionnaires are not extracting specific information from patients and the general format of the tools are not relevant to a particular treatment with a particular disease.

Selection of tools for research is dependent on the researcher's question. For example, in the case of venous leg ulcers, healing of wounds is dependent on several factors, and those that are identified by the present authors are shown in *Figure 8.1*. Hence the choice of tool should cover those factors that affect the patients.

The fish-bone diagram illustrates the potential causes that could affect the healing of chronic venous ulcers. The four primary factors that affect the healing of venous leg ulcers are: the patient; the nurse; the wound; and the dressing material. The labelled arrows represent sub-factors related to each primary factor. The arrow heads provide input towards each factor leading to the central arrow. The central arrow along with the four primary factors contribute to the healing progress of the wound. Under patient factors, age, sex, mobility, tolerance, compliance with the treatment and discomfort experienced are highlighted as the main areas of concern contributing to effective healing.

It is well known that ambulation is required to accelerate the venous return to the heart, aided by the compression bandages (Moneta *et al*, 2000). There were reports that in the younger generation of the population, men suffer from venous ulcers more than women. The latter are more susceptible to the condition in older age than men. Hence, age and sex were included in *Figure 8.1* (Franks and Moffat, 1998). Finally, tolerance and compliance with the compression therapy are required to complete the treatment period.

Nurses who have responsibility for treating patients with venous ulcers need to be aware of the dressing techniques, dressing performance and the need to update their awareness regarding the effective measurement of the wound. Treatment of the wound by the nurse and maintenance of treatment by the patient are other factors that contribute to effective healing. Identifying the chronicity of wounds, their position and applying the correct type of dressing — primary contact layers and secondary dressing with an appropriate bandaging technique — are necessary to the healing process. This needs an effective training and skills to apply the device with adequate knowledge on the part of the nurse.

Figure 8.1 shows the relationship between the problem and possible causes. This helps us to know the factors that are likely to affect the healing process and how they should be addressed in the questionnaires while surveying the perspectives of patients and their health. The primary purpose of measuring health improvements of patients in clinical trials evaluating efficacy of treatment devices is to evaluate the trend of the patients' health over a certain period. These surveys complement the objective clinical evidence obtained in trials. Although a combination of generic and disease-specific questionnaires can be used, lengthy questionnaires are time-consuming and can be tiresome to patients.

Regarding the venous leg ulcer patients, a questionnaire is required to address the need to: measure pain during the treatment; monitor patient ambulation while in treatment; assess patient tolerance to the treatment; investigate patient discomfort owing to compression bandage; study patient compliance to the medical device or therapy; and investigate how medical devices will influence the treatment.

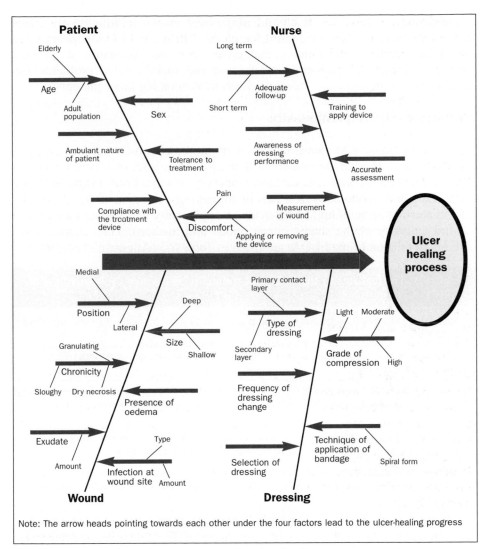

Figure 8.1: Contributory factors to venous leg ulcer healing.

Which questionnaire to use

The focus of the choice of tool is directed on the disease-specific measurement tools: Hyland new tool; CWIS; Charing Cross venous ulcer questionnaire; FLQA; and CIVIQ. Clinical trials were conducted on leg ulcer patients using CWIS and CIVIQ, confirming the usability and relative confidence in using the newly developed questionnaire in clinical trials. However, in the case of Hyland tool, FLQA and Charing Cross leg ulcer questionnaire, no studies were reported using those new tools apart from the validation studies mentioned previously.

Quality of life is a multidimensional construct and covers issues concerning leg ulcer patients, experiences, such as general health, physical functioning, physical symptoms, toxic effects, emotional functioning, social and occupational functioning. It should also cover issues relating to treatment modalities used in trials evaluating biomedical devices. FLQA appears to be the most detailed questionnaire that covers not only domains of physical problems, emotional problems, satisfaction and social related problems, but also discusses the issues of therapy related to venous leg ulcer patients.

Features of FLQA questionnaire

FLQA is a closed-end questionnaire with multiple choice options given to respondents to provide opinion about their QoL from a set of ordered variables (never, rarely, sometimes moderately and very much). Four visual analogue scales help to generate numerical data in domains of pain, general health, venous illness and condition of leg, and provide an opportunity to compute measures of central tendency of the scores (mean, mode and median). The claims of the authors in relation to the FLQA are listed in *Table 8.5* (Augustin *et al*, 1997).

Table 8.5: The features of the FLQA questionnaire as claimed by Augustin *et al* (1997)
Applicable to the adult and elderly patient population as it covers issues that are important to their life
Reliability of individual scales is very high with respect to internal consistency except in therapy and social life
When administered to patients at a two-time period (a month separation) the questionnaire was found to be easily understood in most of the cases and the rate of missing data was less than 5%
Able to discriminate differences between severely affected venous ulcer patients and mildly affected patients. Thus, the questionnaire possesses discriminant validity
The tool is able to detect the effects of treatment and therapy given to patients when followed for three months from start of therapy; this indicates that it is able to assess the change in the patient's condition, showing sensitivity to change
Takes an average of twenty-one minutes to complete and the survey period per patient is not too long. Any survey that takes more than thirty minutes is considered to be a tedious survey (Survey Process, 2001)

Conclusion

Clinical trials in wound care are conducted to evaluate the efficacy and effectiveness of new medical devices on patients. The most important aspect in clinical trials is to assess the impact of treatment device on patients' wellbeing. This helps in the decision-making process in relation to a particular therapy or device. Subjective measurements such as QoL, when coupled with objective measures, broaden the existing knowledge on patients' state of wellbeing and, in turn, contribute to improved health care. Health-related quality of life is a multidimensional concept and it is being measured using generic or disease-specific questionnaires.

Generic measurement tools are more detailed in their coverage on QoL and have broad application on different outcomes and treatments. In contrast, the disease-specific questionnaires are used to measure the impact of certain disease on patients' health. Specific measures are responsive to change and are user-friendly, but cannot be used in different diseases and interventions as generic measures.

A most difficult task is to select a suitable questionnaire that has already been shown to possess an acceptable level of validity, reliability and responsiveness, and that discusses the problems experienced by venous-ulcerated patients and issues relating to compression therapy. While selecting the suitable tool for assessing the HRQoL in clinical trials it is necessary to be familiar with the disease, study population and factors that affect the venous ulcer healing process. Researchers who have used generic tools in their studies recommend the use of disease-specific or ulcer-specific questionnaires, as generic questionnaire are much broader and not specific to the venous ulcer patients.

The FLQA, whose features have been outlined earlier, is found to possess all the required features that are of interest for implementation in clinical trials for evaluating the patients' QoL. Hence, FLQA, along with the additional factors relating to venous leg ulcers as cited previously, will be a complete survey tool that will allow the researcher to assess the perspectives of patients on their general health and medical devices, and overall QoL issues while conducting clinical trials in wound care.

Health-related quality of life measurements in venous leg ulcerated patients can be a tremendous value in the management of patients, in making necessary changes in the treatment and relevant characteristics of medical devices when using such a disease-specific venous leg ulcer questionnaire.

Key points

- ⌘ The evidence base for wound care practice is deficient without the patients' perspective.

- ⌘ Disease-specific venous leg ulcer questionnaires are more pertinent and appropriate to venous-ulcerated patients than generic tools.

- ⌘ Recently developed venous ulcer-specific tools should be carefully selected and implemented in clinical trials because the use of newly developed disease-specific venous ulcer questionnaires have not been reported in clinical trials evaluating medical devices.

- ⌘ Factors that influence the venous ulcer healing process are the patient, nurse, wound and dressing material. The supplementary items that need to be added are patient ambulation, tolerance, discomfort, compliance, and overall influence of the treatment.

References

Augustin M, Dieterle W, Zschocke I *et al* (1997) Development and validation of a disease-specific questionnaire on the quality of life of patients with chronic venous insufficiency. *J Vasc Dis* **26**: 291–301

Bale S, Vanessa J, Balliére T (1997) *Principles of Wound Interventions, Wound Care Nursing, A Patient-centred Approach*. Baillière Tindall, London

Bennett G, Moody M (1995) *Wound Care for Health Professionals*. Chapman & Hall, London

Bullinger M, Kirchberger I, von Steinbuchel N (1993) Der gregebogen Alltagsleben — ein Verfahren zur Erfassung der gesundheitsbezogenen Lebensqualitat. *Z Med Psychol* **3**: 212–31

Callam MJ, Harper DR, Dale JJ, Ruckley CV (1987) Chronic ulcer of leg: clincal history. *Br Med J* **294**: 1391

de Charro F (2001) Euroqol questionnaire, Euroqol group, Dr Frank de Charro, Euroqol Business Manager, The Netherlands, EQ-5D www.euroqol.org

Fayers PM, Machin D (2000) *Quality of Life Assessment, Analysis and Interpretation*. John Wiley and Son, Chichester

Franks PJ, Moffat CJ (1998) Who suffers most from leg ulceration? *J Wound Care* **7**(8): 383–5

Franks PJ, Moffat CJ, Ellison DA (1999) Quality of life in venous ulceration: A randomized trial of two bandage systems. *Phlebology* **14**(3): 95–9

Holbrock M, Skilbeck C (1983) An activities index for use with stroke patients. *Age Ageing* **12**: 166–70

Hunt SM, McEwen J, McKenna SP (1984) Perceived health: age and sex comparisons in the community. *J Epidemiol Community Health* **38**: 156–60

Hunt SM, McEven J, McKenna SP (1985) Measuring health status: a new tool for clinicians and epidemiologists. *J R Coll Gen Pract* **35**: 185–8

Hyland ME, Thompson B (1994) Quality of life of leg ulcer patients: questionnaire and preliminary findings. *J Wound Care* **3**(6): 294–8

Jenkinson C, Coulter A, Wright L (1993) Short form (SF-36) health survey questionnaire; normative data for adults of working age. *Br Med J* **306**: 1437–40

Launois R, Reboul-Marty J, Henry B (1996) Construction and validation of a quality of life questionnaire in chronic lower limb venous insufficiency (CIVIQ). *Qual Life Res* **5**: 539–54

Lindholm C, Bjellerup M, Christensen OB *et al* (1993) Quality of life in chronic leg ulcers. *Acta Derm Venerol* **73**: 440–3

Marlow S (1999) System 4: the four-layer bandage system from SSL International. *Br J Nurs* **8**(16): 1104–7

Mayberry JC, Moneta GL, Taylor LM, Porter JM (1991) Fifteen year results of ambulatory compression therapy for chronic venous ulcers. *Surgery* **109**: 571–81

Melzack R (1975) The McGill pain questionnaire, major properties and scoring methods. *Pain* **1**: 277–99

Moneta GL, Nicoloff AD, Porter JM (2000) Compression treatment of chronic venous ulceration: a review. *Phlebology* **15**: 162–8

Morison M, Moffat C, Nixon JB, Bale S (1998) *A Colour Guide to Nursing Management of Chronic Wounds*. 2nd edn. Jill Northcott, London

Nelzén O (2000) Leg ulcers: economic aspects. *Phlebology* **15**: 110–14

Price P (1993) Defining quality of life. *J Wound Care* **2**(5): 304–6

Price PE (1998) Health-related quality of life and patients' perspectives. *J Wound Care* **7**(7): 365–6

Price PE, Harding KG (1996) Measuring health-related quality of life in patients with chronic leg ulcers. *WOUNDS: A Compendium of Clinical Research and Practice* **8**(3): 91–4

Price PE, Harding K (1997) The suitability of a wound specific QoL measure (CWIS) for patients with diabetes-related foot ulcers. Presentation to ETRS, Cologne, Germany (available from The British Library, Boston Spa, Wetherby, West Yorkshire, UK)

Price PE, Harding KG (2000) Acute and chronic wounds: differences in self-reported health-related quality of life. *J Wound Care* **9**(2): 93–5

Reid J (1996) Quality of life measurement tools. *J Wound Care* **5**(3): 142

Smith JJ, Guest MG, Greenhalgh MA, Davies AH (2000) Measuring the quality of life in patients with venous ulcers. *J Vasc Surg* **31**: 642–9

Survey Process (2001) US General Services Administration, Office of Government Wide Policy, FirstGov, Washington DC, USA (www.itpolicy. sa.gov/mkm/pathways/survey/scoop14.htm)

Thomas C (2001) *Management of the Patient with a Venous Ulcer, Advances in Skin and Wound Care.* Williams & Wilkins, Springhouse, USA

Vayssairat M, Ziani E, Houot B (2000) Placebo controlled efficacy of class I stockings in chronic venous insufficiency of the lower limbs. *J Mal Vasc* **25**(4): 256–62

Venkatraman P, Anand S, Dean C, Nettleton R (2002a) Clinical trials in wound care I: advantages and limitations of different clinical trial designs. *J Wound Care* **11**(3): 91–4

Venkatraman P, Anand S, Dean C, Nettleton R (2002b) Clinical trials in wound care II: achieving statistical significance. *J Wound Care* **11**(4): 156–160

Veraat JCJM, Pronk G, Neuman HAM (1997a) Pressure differences of elastic compression stockings at the ankle region. *Dermatol Surg* **23**: 935–9

Veraat JCJM, Daaman E, de Vet HCW (1997b) Elastic compression stockings' durability of pressure in daily practice. *Vasa* **26**: 282–6

Walters SJ, Morell CJ, Dixon S (1999) Measuring health-related quality of life in patients with venous leg ulcers. *Qual Life Res* **8**: 327–6

Ware JJ, Sherbourne CD (1992) The MOS 36-item short form health survey (SF-36), conceptual framework and item selection. *J Med Care* **30**: 473–83

World Health Organization (1976) *Basic Documents.* WHO, Geneva: 1

World Health Organization (1984) *Uses of Epidemiology in Ageing, Report of a Scientific Group, 1983.* Technical Report Series. WHO, Geneva: 706

Zimmet SE (1999) Venous leg ulcers: modern evaluation and management. *Dermatol Surg* **25**: 236–41

9

Compromised wound healing: a scientific approach to treatment

Keith Moore

A well-defined sequence of events follow dermal injury and with normal healing there is a controlled progression to re-epithelialization, scarring and restoration of an intact epidermis. In contrast, compromised wounds such as diabetic ulcers, varicose ulcers and decubitus ulcers fail to heal and if not given appropriate care will enlarge and may persist for many months or even years. Our knowledge of healing has grown significantly since Winter's pioneering demonstration that maintenance of a moist wound environment would assist healing (Winter, 1962). This observation stimulated development of wound dressings with physical properties designed to maintain an optimum level of wound moisture while still removing excess exudate and acting as a barrier to infection. Understanding of the cell biology and biochemistry of healing and non-healing wounds gained over the following four decades has allowed characterisation of the healing process and the defects that develop in compromised wounds. This growing body of knowledge is leading to the rational design of treatments for chronic wounds that interact with the cellular environment to modulate the healing process with the intention of stimulating healing.

Differences between normally healing and compromised wounds

Normal wound healing

Haemostasis is promoted rapidly after injury when platelets released from blood at the wound site bind to freshly exposed tissue components. These cells contain many chemicals that act as messenger molecules responsible for initiating blood coagulation, inflammation and wound healing. For healing, one of the most important molecules released is platelet-derived growth factor (PDGF) which attracts neutrophils and monocytes from the blood and fibroblasts from adjacent dermis into the wound site by a process known as chemotaxis. These cells then initiate the healing process. The importance of PDGF is emphasized by the fact that it was one of the first pharmaceutical products developed as a wound treatment from our knowledge of the healing process and is now available for topical application to enhance wound healing (Nagai, 2002).

Inflammation following injury is a normal part of healing but it rapidly resolves and is followed by a cell proliferation phase. Fibroblasts at the wound site are stimulated by PDGF and other growth factors to proliferate and produce extracellular matrix (ECM) as a component of granulation tissue. The presence of functional ECM is required to allow keratinocyte migration from the wound edge and re-epithelialize the wound surface with eventual scar formation.

Many growth factors and other proteins known as cytokines are involved in regulating the healing process (Moore, 2001). They are synthesized by all cell types present and, once released in an active form, bind to receptors on other cells to control their activity. This raises the possibility that they may be used for therapeutic interventions as demonstrated for PDGF. Conversely, because they act in complex networks any disruption to the network may delay healing.

Compromised wounds

A common feature of compromised wounds is that they appear arrested at the stage of inflammation and granulation tissue formation (*Table 9.1*). Non-resolution of inflammation and the presence of bacteria (Trengrove *et al*, 1996) results in generation of wound exudates containing a disordered cytokine/growth factor network and high levels of proteolytic enzymes (proteases) that destroy tissue proteins, growth factors and ECM (*Table 9.2*) (Brantigan, 1996). Because the ECM is degraded proliferating keratinocytes at the wound margin cannot migrate over the wound bed to achieve wound closure.

Table 9.1: Differences in cell activity between healing and compromised wounds

Normal healing	Compromised healing
Haemostasis Platelet aggregation/factor release	**Chronic inflammation** Infection/bacterial colonisation Neutrophil accumulation
Early inflammation Neutrophil accumulation and decrease	Inappropriate macrophage and lymphocyte populations High protease levels
Late inflammation Monocyte/lymphocyte accumulation and decrease	Inappropriate growth factors/cytokines
	Granulation tissue formation Continuing fibroblast proliferation
Granulation tissue formation Fibroblast/endothelial cell proliferation	Inappropriate ECM Endothelial cell proliferation Tortuous blood vessel formation
Extracellular matrix formation	**Degraded extracellular matrix**
Re-epithelialization Keratinocyte proliferation and migration	**Re-epithelialization** Defective/inhibited keratinocyte migration

Proteases

The majority of cell types present in wound tissue have the capacity to produce proteases and normally both their secretion and proteolytic activity is tightly controlled. Proteases are required to destroy necrotic tissue, temporarily break down ECM to allow cell and capillary migration and to remodel ECM in scar tissue so that it achieves maximum strength. However, in compromised wounds there is a shortage of regulatory factors that act to inhibit protease activity as well as an overproduction of proteases. Additionally, many compromised wounds are contaminated with bacteria that also have the ability to add to the pool of proteases in the wound. For instance, *Pseudomonas aeruginosa*, which is found in 20–30% of venous leg ulcers can secrete both elastases and proteases to disrupt healing (Schmidtchen *et al*, 2001). The resulting overall loss of control of protease activity has great potential to compromise the healing process.

Table 9.2: Bioactivity of wound exudate from healing and compromised wounds

Healing wound	Compromised wound
Stimulates	**Inhibits**
Angiogenesis	Endothelial cell proliferation
Fibroplasia	Fibroblast proliferation
Collagen synthesis	Keratinocyte proliferation
Contains	Collagen synethesis
Epidermal growth factor	Contains elevated protease levels
Fibroblast growth factor	**Degrades**
Platelet-derived growth factor	Growth factors
Transforming growth factor	Extracellular matrix components

Growth factors and extracellular matrix (ECM)

Increased protease activity in compromised wounds results in degradation of growth factors (Yager, 1997) needed for regulation of healing and destruction of ECM (Grinnell and Zhu, 1996).

Extracellular matrix is primarily manufactured by fibroblasts in the skin and interlaced fibres of the proteins, collagen and elastin, produce its structural strength and elasticity. Other specialized proteins, such as fibronectin and laminin, with a combination of proteins and polysaccharides known as proteoglycans are found in various combinations depending on wound age. While the mechanical properties of ECM are important for skin function it is clear that ECM also plays a major role in regulating healing by acting as a reservoir for growth factors to be called on when required during healing (Appleton *et al,* 1993). Additionally, ECM components such as fibronectin or vitronectin bind to keratinocytes and induce them to migrate over granulation tissue as part of wound re-epithelialization (O'Toole, 2001).

Destruction of ECM by uncontrolled proteases is considered to be a major contributory factor preventing healing of compromised wounds (Fray *et al*, 2003). Protease activity is a good example of how intrinsic factors required for normal healing (Steffenson *et al*, 2001) negatively impact on healing when acting in an uncontrolled manner outside normal regulatory circuits. This leads to the concept that restoration of normal regulation will induce healing (Schultz *et al*, 2003).

Potential therapeutic approaches to treatment of intrinsic defects in chronic wounds

Conventional wound therapies tend to focus on dealing with extrinsic factors that have a negative impact on healing. Glycaemic control and offloading the affected foot with diabetic foot ulcers, compression therapy to treat vascular disease in venous leg ulcers and pressure relief for decubitus ulcers. Whilst these measures will induce healing of many chronic wounds a significant proportion will fail to heal or only heal slowly (Franks *et al*, 1995).

The growing body of knowledge of chronic wound biology allows for a rational approach to develop new treatments. Initiation of healing a chronic wound intuitively requires conversion of the chronic healing status to that of a healing acute wound. This concept is supported by evidence at the molecular level from those wounds that respond to conventional therapies. For example, the cytokine profiles of wound fluid taken from leg ulcers responding to compression therapy change from angiostatic to angiogenic cytokines whilst those representing the inflammatory state indicate a change from a chronic to resolving inflammation as might be seen in an acute wound (Fivenson *et al*, 1997). Studies of this type characterising the cell and molecular biology of the chronic wound state have identified a number of intrinsic factors as potential targets for therapy (*Figure 9.1*).

Infection and inflammation

The pathological significance of the presence of bacteria within wound tissue and its impact on healing is controversial. Even healing chronic wounds tend to be colonised with a number of microorganisms and a continuum extends from colonisation to infection, with a laboratory-based definition of infection being difficult to achieve (Bowler *et al*, 2001). It is without doubt that clinical infection will delay healing when the number of colonising species increases (Trengove *et al*, 1996) and the total bioburden passes threshold values thought to be greater than 10^5 organisms/gm of tissue (Robson, 1997), although for *b-haemolytic Streptococci* the threshold may be as low as 10^3 for impairment of healing. Regardless of a precise definition of infection, it is clear that granulation tissue of most chronic wounds will be exposed to bacteria in some degree. Bacteria can interact with the healing process in a number of different ways. They may produce molecular species (virulence factors) such as proteases that directly affect the healing process or bioactive molecules such as lipopolysaccharide (LPS or endotoxin) that are potent stimulators of inflammatory cells. Additionally, when phagocytosed as part of the innate inflammatory response to infection they will stimulate macrophages and neutrophils to synthesise and release pro-inflammatory cytokines and proteases.

Elimination of bacteria from the wound environment is clearly desirable from a number of different perspectives and this objective provides an immediate therapeutic target. Efforts to restrict indiscriminate antibiotic use and prevent development of bacterial antibiotic resistance has driven the development of wound dressings that deliver antibacterials which minimise the risk of resistance. The latest generation of which utilise silver formulations with the advantage of antibacterial activity at the wound site with minimal systemic effects and reduce toxicity. These dressings can be multi-functional and manage odour and exudate simultaneously (White, 2003).

Whilst antibacterials may be used to treat infected wounds they are unlikely to be used for prophylaxis of colonised wounds without signs of infection, so the situation remains that most chronic wounds will have some level of bacterial bioburden interacting with the healing process. The consequence of persisting low levels of bacteria in the wound is an accumulation of bacterial products and prolonged stimulation of inflammation. This is a contributing factor to high levels of protease activity and a disordered cytokine and growth factor profile found in compromised wounds.

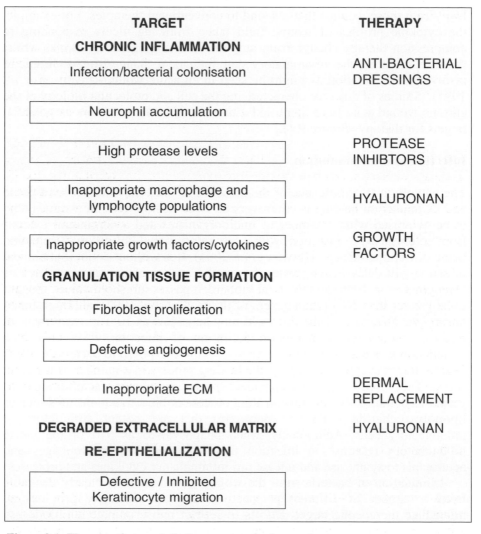

Figure 9.1: Therapeutic targets in the compromised wound

Proteases

It is well documented that chronic wounds exhibit elevated protease levels compared to healing acute wounds (Agren, 1994). Protease activity is regulated in part by naturally occurring inhibitors known as TIMPs (tissue inhibitor of metalloprotease) and the levels of these are reduced in chronic wound exudate (Bullen, 1995). As venous leg ulcers (VLU) heal in response to compression therapy, levels of matrix metalloproteases (MMPs) decrease. In chronic wounds MMP levels may be thirty-fold higher than in acute wounds (Trengove,1999). Assuming that this change is not an epi-phenomenon then reduction of protease levels may make an attractive therapeutic target which, if treated, would prevent ECM destruction and aid re-epithelialisation.

This rationale is one of the proposed mechanisms of action of a new dressing marketed as a protease modulating matrix, for the treatment of compromised wounds. It is composed of a mixture of freeze dried cellulose and oxidised regenerated cellulose (Cullen, 2002a) and, in addition to inactivating proteases in wound exudate (Cullen, 2002b), also acts to bind growth factors and protect them from proteolytic degradation (Clark *et al*, 2002). Evidence of clinical efficacy for this dressing has been demonstrated by an accelerated rate of decrease in VLU wound area of 55% in eight weeks treatment compared to a control group decrease of 36% (Vin *et al*, 2002).

An alternative means of achieving protease inhibition is to use pharmacologically active compounds that target these enzymes. There is currently interest in this type of compound because of the potential therapeutic application for treatment of a number of diseases including rheumatoid arthritis and cancer metastasis (Rudek *et al*, 2002). This approach may also prove valuable in treatment of chronic wounds. However, although proteases play a role in the pathogenesis of chronic wounds they also have a role to play in normal healing with involvement in autolytic debridement, cell migration and ECM re-modelling. Their levels are elevated early after injury and rapidly decrease in the absence of infection but activity is still detectable in normal human surgical wounds six days post-operatively (Tarlton, 1999). Thus, it may not be desirable to induce total protease inhibition to achieve healing. One approach may be to use highly specific protease inhibitors so that only those enzymes associated with non-healing are inhibited, whilst those associated with healing are unaffected. This property has recently been ascribed to a synthetic compound which targets MMP-3 mediated ECM degradation whilst leaving those enzymes associated with cell migration unaffected (Fray *et al*, 2003).

Growth factors

The paradigm that normal healing is regulated by the co-ordinate actions of cytokine growth factors and that such regulation is disordered in the chronic wound led to the concept that intervention with exogenous growth factors may stimulate healing (Bennett and Schultz, 1993). Implementation of this strategy was made possible by the availability of an increasing number of recombinant human growth factors with functions known to be important in healing. Key examples that have been evaluated in human clinical studies are presented below.

Platelet-derived growth factor (PDGF)

Platelet-derived growth factor plays a central role to initiate healing after its release from platelets aggregating at the site of tissue injury. It acts as a chemoattractant stimulating the directed migration of neutrophils, macrophages and fibroblasts; it activates macrophages to synthesise and release other growth factors and stimulates production of fibronectin, hyaluronan and proteases by fibroblasts. Early studies of treatment of DFU with platelet releasate indicated accelerated wound closure by comparison to placebo (Steed, 1992). Platelet releasate is essentially the cytoplasmic contents of homologous platelets and whilst containing PDGF also contains other growth factors such as EGF, TGF and FGF (Steed, 1992). However, the beneficial effect of topically applied recombinant PDGF was later confirmed in treatment of DFU (Steed, 1995). In this twenty-week study, 48% of wounds treated with PDGF achieved complete wound healing compared to 25% in the placebo group, with mean 98.8% and 82.1% wound area reductions in each group respectively. Recombinant PDGF has been licensed for treatment of DFU and whilst not 100% effective in all cases has been demonstrated in cost effectiveness analyses to result in twenty-six fewer ulcer days per patient (Sibbald *et al*, 2003).

Granulocyte-monocyte colony stimulating factor (GM-CSF)

GM-CSF is produced by T-lymphocytes and macrophages following their activation. It was originally named because it was found to stimulate proliferation of granulocyte and monocyte progenitor cells. As with most growth factors it is multifunctional and, in the context of wound healing, those properties that may be important include attraction and differentiation of neutrophils and macrophages with a consequential enhancement of their microbicidal capacity. It is an important mediator for regulation of inflammatory responses and synergises with other cytokines. Additionally, it is chemotactic for keratinocytes, modulates fibroblast function and stimulates endothelial proliferation.

With such an impressive array of healing related effects, it is not surprising that GM-CSF has been evaluated for the treatment of human chronic wounds. As with other growth factors a positive effect was found but no study has demonstrated a result approaching 100% efficacy. Subsets of refractory chronic wounds have been demonstrated to respond rapidly (Malik *et al*, 1998); an improvement from 19% of placebo to 57% or 61% healed VLU depending on GM-CSF dose (Da Costa *et al*, 1999).

Transforming growth factor beta (TGF-ß)

Transforming growth factor beta exists as three isoform (TGF-ß1, TGF-ß2, TGF-ß3) and can be produced by all cells in the wound environment, suggesting a multiplicity of functions, including chemotaxis of leucocytes and stimulation of angiogenesis. Additionally, it is essential for wound maturation and strength as it stimulates fibroblast production of collagen, fibronectin and glycosaminoglycans. These properties led to its proposal as a wound healing agent (Amento and Beck, 1991). Published evidence of efficacy in chronic wounds is limited although there is some evidence of an early stimulation of healing in pressure ulcers. However, this effect did not result in a difference in overall healing rates compared to placebo at the end of a sixteen-week study (Hirshberg, 2001). There is some evidence that TGF-ß2 may accelerate normal incisional healing (Wright *et al*, 2000) and act synergistically with PDGF in healing experimental diabetic wounds (Brown *et al*, 1994).

Keratinocyte growth factor-2 (KGF-2)

Keratinocyte growth factor-2 is a member of the fibroblast growth factor family (FGF-10). It is synthesised by fibroblasts and stimulates proliferation of the majority of keratinocytes. This mode of action has been demonstrated to accelerate healing in animal models of normal (Soler *et al*, 1999) and impaired (Xia *et al*, 1999) healing. Application to human wounds did not demonstrate such a positive effect with little difference between KGF-2 treated and placebo in numbers of VLU achieving closure within twelve weeks. However, an increased rate of area decrease was observed in the KGF-2 group with the treatment being more effective with long standing smaller ulcers (Robson *et al*, 2001).

A partial response to therapy after application of a single type of growth factor is not surprising considering that healing follows a temporal sequence of growth factor gene expression. It may be that optimal dosing regimens will have to be derived that apply different combinations of growth factors in an appropriate order (Robson *et al*, 2000). Proteolytic degradation of applied growth factors may also negate their effect and it has been suggested that there may be a requirement for co-administration of a protease inhibitor to protect the therapeutic agent (Trengove *et al*, 1999). Finally, to compensate for the heterogeneity of response to growth factor therapy, consideration has to be given to development of a diagnostic system that will predict the appropriate factor(s) requirement for each wound.

Bioengineered dermal replacements

Autologous skin grafts taken using split thickness or pinch grafting have been used successfully to treat chronic wounds. They suffer from a number of disadvantages in terms of availability of donor sites, patient discomfort on creation of a second wound site and possible scarring (Valencia *et al*, 2000). Developments in the fields of biomaterials and *in vitro* tissue expansion has allowed development of the new discipline of bioengineering. This technology has produced a number of products intended to replace autologous skin grafts with a standardised off-the-shelf product for treatment of non-healing ulcers. Such dermal replacements are essentially comprised of a biocompatible, bio-resorbable scaffold that acts as a carrier to cultured fibroblasts, keratinocytes or both. In addition to covering the wound, they act as a donor of cells and growth factors to the wound site.

Two products have been evaluated in some depth for the treatment of chronic wounds. One of these, Dermagraft™ , uses a polygalactin scaffold with cultured human neonatal fibroblasts. Whilst the cells proliferate during the manufacturing process they synthesise an extracellular matrix composed of collagen, glycosaminoglycans and fibronectin which acts as a reservoir for synthesised growth factors. It is thought to be a particularly active stimulator of angiogenesis in the recipient wound (Roberts and Mansbridge, 2002). The efficacy of Dermagraft™ treatment was compared to conventional DFU treatment in a multi-centre US study. Assessed by the endpoint of wound closure by week twelve of treatment, 30% of the Dermagraft™ group healed compared to 18.3% of the controls (Marston *et al*, 2003).

The second product, Apligraf™ , is more complex in that it is a bilayered skin equivalent with dermal (fibroblast) and epidermal (keratinocyte) components. The first layer fibroblasts are cultured for six days on a semi-permeable membrane with bovine collagen to form a dermal matrix. This is then seeded with keratinocytes which proliferate and differentiate into an epidermal layer that is allowed to mature and form a stratum corneum (Streit and Braathen, 2000). In effect, the product is a viable skin construct and has been used to treat VLU and DFU with some success. Treatment of DFU produced an increase in those healed from 38 to 56% with a median reduction in healing time from ninety to sixty-five days. With VLU an increase from 49 to 63% healing was observed in those treated with Apligraf™ plus compression therapy compared to compression alone (Curran and Plosker, 2002).

As with growth factor treatment, 100% response was not seen with these therapies emphasizing the requirement for a means of identifying those patients likely to respond to treatment. This is particularly important when the relatively high cost of these products is considered.

Extracellular matrix (ECM)

Extracellular matrix is composed of a mixture of collagen and elastin fibrils that provide strength and elasticity to skin. These proteins are co-mingled with proteoglycans which are protein-carbohydrate complexes characterised by their glycosaminoglycan (GAG) component. GAGs are highly charged sulphated and carboxylated polyanionic linear polysaccharides. Those most commonly present within the ECM are hyaluronan (HA), chondroitin Sulphate, dermatan sulphate, heparan sulphate and keratan sulphate.

Hyaluronan (HA), previously known as hyaluronic acid, consists of alternating glucuronic acid and N-acetylglucosamine units. It is synthesised by fibroblasts and is a major component of wound ECM, and because of its high level of hydration confers viscosity to tissues and fluids. Its physicochemical properties modulate cell functions by acting as a hygroscopic osmotic buffer, by its chemical properties such as free radical scavenging, anti-oxidant effects and its ability to exclude enzymes from the local cellular environment. Additionally, it may interact directly with cells via the RHAMM receptor (receptor for HA mediated motility), the CD44 receptor and the ICAM-1 (inter-cellular adhesion molecule-1) receptor. Receptor interaction may be via a ligand receptor type interaction (CD44) or via a receptor blockade (ICAM-1) (Chen and Abatangelo, 1999).

Hyaluronan potentially plays a role in each phase of healing. During the inflammatory phase of healing wound tissue is rich in HA. It may play multiple roles, promoting inflammation early in healing by enhancing leucocyte infiltration and also moderating the inflammatory response as healing progresses towards granulation tissue formation.

Granulation tissue is also rich in HA and here its role includes facilitation of cell migration (fibroblasts and endothelial cells) into the provisional matrix. Although HA has not been demonstrated to be mitogenic, its oligosaccharide derivatives do stimulate endothelial cell proliferation (West and Kumar, 1989).

Hyaluronan is present in high concentrations in the basal layer of the epidermis in normal skin and co-localises with the CD44 receptor expressed by keratinocytes migrating over the provisional matrix of wound granulation tissue. Suppression of CD44 expression and consequential decreased HA binding results in defective inflammatory responses, decreased skin elasticity and impaired healing.

Hyaluronan applied to the wound surface absorbs wound exudate to create a gel forming a HA rich moist wound environment that has been demonstrated to stimulate healing in human chronic wounds (Ortonne, 1996), and wound dressings are now available manufactured from the benzyl ester of HA. This slows down degradation by introducing the requirement for de-esterification to provide a slow release of HA into the wound environment (Benedetti *et al*, 1993). Treatment with this product has been demonstrated to produce a higher degree of wound closure for indolent neuropathic ulcers (Edmonds and Foster, 2000) and a pilot study of twenty VLU indicates that it will promote healing of this lesion as 4/20 healed at eight weeks of treatment, and the remaining ulcers achieved a mean area reduction of 53% in wound area (Colleta *et al*, 2003).

Conclusion

Historically, wound dressings made from readily available absorbent materials such as cotton were easily sterilised and relatively inexpensive. They were used with the major objectives of absorbing blood and exudate and assisting with infection control. Their major disadvantage was that they did not satisfy the requirement for a moist wound environment demonstrated to be necessary for optimal healing in the 1960s. Following this discovery a range of materials were introduced that were selected for their fluid handling properties to achieve a moist wound environment. Some of the dressing components, such as alginates (Thomas, 2000) were subsequently found to exert a bioactivity that possibly affects the healing process. These properties were not deliberately engineered into wound management products but this is now an achievable objective.

One of the most difficult challenges for laboratory scientists is to translate their theoretical knowledge into a practical reality that is of use to both the practitioner and the patient. The advanced therapies described above demonstrate how understanding defects within the chronic wound (*Table 9.1*) has allowed definition of therapeutic targets (*Figure 9.1*) and development of appropriate modes of treatment. The linkage of various factors also indicates how an appropriate choice of target will rectify multiple defects.

Advanced therapies tend to be more expensive than conventional treatments and are likely to be used for non-responsive wounds. All the studies evaluating these treatments demonstrate that they are only effective in a subset of patients and indiscriminate use will lead to unnecessary expense. This, in turn, requires development of diagnostic systems that will identify appropriate therapies for individual patients.

Our knowledge of the cell biology of wound healing now allows for the rationale design of wound management products that will stimulate healing of compromised wounds, such as diabetic ulcers and venous leg ulcers. This process has been demonstrated by the development of recently introduced products that represent a new generation of bioactive therapies that will interact with various phases of the healing process and enhance our ability to treat compromised wounds.

Key points

⌘ Increased understanding of the cellular and molecular biology of normal healing and the defects that arise in compromised wounds has allowed development of a new generation of bioactive wound therapies.

⌘ Compromised wounds such as diabetic ulcers, decubitus ulcers and venous leg ulcers exhibit chronic inflammation, high protease levels, growth factor defects and degraded extracellular matrix.

⌘ Conventional dressings generate an optimal wound moisture level but are not designed to treat other defects found in compromised wounds.

⌘ New wound management products have been developed to stimulate healing of compromised wounds by modulating inflammation, delivering growth factors or inhibiting protease activity.

References

Agren MS (1994) Gelatinase activity during wound healing. *Br J Dermatol* **131**: 634–40

Amento EP, Beck LS (1991) TGF-beta and wound healing. *Ciba Found Symp* **157**: 115–23

Appleton I, Tomlinson A, Colville-Nash PR, Willoughby DA (1993) Temporal and spatial immunolocalization of cytokines in murine chronic granulomatous tissue. Implications for their role in tissue development and repair processes. *Lab Invest* **69**: 405–14

Bowler PG, Duerden BI, Armstrong DG (2001) Wound microbiology and associated approaches to wound management. *Clin Microbiol Rev* **14**: 244–69

Benedetti L, Cortivo R, Berti T *et al* (1993) Biocompatibility and biodegradation of different hyaluronan derivatives (Hyaff) implanted in rats. *Biomaterials* **14**: 1154–60

Bennett NT, Schultz GS (1993) Growth factors and wound healing: Part II. Role in normal and chronic wound healing. *Am J Surg* **166**: 74–81

Brantigan CO (1996) The history of the understanding of growth factors in wound healing. *Wounds* **8**: 78–90

Brown RL, Breeden MP, Greenhalgh DG (1994) PDGF and TGF-alpha act synergistically to improve wound healing in the genetically diabetic mouse. *J Surg Res* **56**: 562–70

Bullen EC, Longaker MT, Updike DL *et al* (1995) Tissue inhibitor of metalloproteases-1 is decreased and activated gelatinases are increased in chronic wounds. *J Invest Dermatol* **104**: 236–40

Chen WY, Abatangclo G (1999) Functions of hyaluronan in wound repair. *Wound Rep Regen* **7**: 79–89

Clark R, Cullen B, McCulloch E, Feng-Yi C (2002) The ability of ORC/collagen to bind, protect and deliver growth factors. Presented at the European Wound Management Association Conference, Granada, Spain

Colletta V, Dioguardi D, Di Lonardo A, Maggio G, Torasso F (2003) A trial to assess the efficacy and tolerability of Hyalofill-F in non-healing venous leg ulcers. *J Wound Care* **12**: 357–60

Cullen B, Watt PW, Lundqvist C *et al* (2002a) The role of oxidized regenerated cellulose/collagen in chronic wound repair and its potential mechanism of action. *Int J Biochem Cell Biol* **34**: 1544–56

Cullen B, Smith R, McCulloch E, Silcocok D, Morrison L (2002b) Mechanism of action of PROMOGRAN, a protease modulating matrix, for the treatment of diabetic foot ulcers. *Wound Rep Regen* **10**: 16–25

Curran, MP, Plosker PL (2002) Bilayered bioengineered skin substitute (Apligraf): a review of its use in the treatment of venous leg ulcers and diabetic foot ulcers. *BioDrugs* **16**: 439–55

Da Costa RM, Ribeiro Jesus FM, Aniceto C, Mendes M (1999) Randomized, double-blind, placebo-controlled, dose-ranging study of granulocyte-macrophage colony stimulating factor in patients with chronic venous leg ulcers. *Wound Rep Regen* **7**: 17–25

Edmonds M , Foster A (2000) Hyalofill: a new product for chronic wound management. *Diab Foot* **3**: 29–30

Fivenson DP, Faria DT, Nickoloff BJ *et al* (1997) Chemokine and inflammatory cytokine changes during chronic wound healing. *Wound Rep Regen* **5**: 310–22

Franks PJ, Moffatt CJ, Connolly M *et al* (1995) Factors associated with healing leg ulceration with high compression. *Age Ageing* **24**: 407–10

Fray MJ, Dickinson RP, Huggins JP, Occleston NL (2003) A potent, selective inhibitor of matrix metalloproteinase-3 for the topical treatment of chronic dermal ulcers. *J Med Chem* **46**: 3514–25

Grinnell F, Zhu M (1996) Fibronectin degradation in chronic wounds depends on the relative levels of elastase, alpha1-proteinase inhibitor, and alpha2-macroglobulin. *J Invest Dermatol* **106**: 335–41

Hirshberg J, Coleman J, Marchant B, Rees RS (2001) TGF-beta3 in the treatment of pressure ulcers: a preliminary report. *Adv Skin Wound Care* **14**: 91–5

Malik IA, Zahid M, Haq S, Syed S, Moid I, Waheed I (1998) Effect of subcutaneous injection of granulocyte-macrophage colony stimulating factor (GM-CSF) on healing of chronic refractory wounds. *Eur J Surg* **164**: 737–44

Marston WA, Hanft J, Norwood P, Pollak R (2003) The efficacy and safety of Dermagraft in improving the healing of chronic diabetic foot ulcers: results of a prospective randomized trial. *Diabetes Care* **26**: 1701–5

Moore K (2001) The scientific basis of wound healing. *Adv Tissue Banking* **5**: 379–97, Pub World Scientific Publishing Co Pte Ltd

Nagai MK, Embil JM (2002) Becaplermin: recombinant platelet derived growth factor, a new treatment for healing diabetic foot ulcers. *Expert Opin Biol Ther* **2**: 211–8

Ortonne JP (1996) A controlled study of the activity of hyaluronic acid in the treatment of venous leg ulcers. *J Dermatol Treat* **7**:75–81

O'Toole EA (2001) Extracellular matrix and keratinocyte migration. *Clin Exp Dermatol* **26**: 525–30

Roberts C, Mansbridge J (2002) The scientific basis and differentiating features of Dermagraft. *Can J Plast Surg* **10** Suppl A: 6A–13A

Robson M (1997) Wound Infection — A failure of wound healing caused by an imbalance of bacteria. *Surg Clin North America* **77**: 637–50

Robson MC, Hill DP, Smith PD *et al* (2000) Sequential cytokine therapy for pressure ulcers: clinical and mechanistic response. *Ann Surg* **231**: 600–11

Robson MC, Phillips TJ, Falanga V *et al* (2001) Randomized trial of topically applied repifermin (recombinant human keratinocyte growth factor-2) to accelerate wound healing in venous ulcers. *Wound Rep Regen* **9**: 347–52

Rudek MA, Venitz J, Figg WD (2002) Matrix metalloproteinase inhibitors: do they have a place in anticancer therapy? *Pharmacotherapy* **22**: 705–20

Schmidtchen A, Wolff H, Hansson C (2001) Differential proteinase expression by *Pseudomonas aeruginosa* derived from chronic leg ulcers. *Acta Derm Venereol* **81**: 406–9

Schultz GS, Sibbald RG, Falanga V *et al* (2003) Wound bed preparation: a systematic approach to wound management. *Wound Rep Regen* **11** (Suppl 1):S1–S28

Sibbald RG, Torrance G, Hux M, Attard C, Milkovich N (2003) Cost-effectiveness of becaplermin for non-healing neuropathic diabetic foot ulcers. *Ostomy Wound Manage* **49**: 76–84

Soler PM, Wright TE, Smith PD *et al* (1999) In vivo characterization of keratinocyte growth factor-2 as a potential wound healing agent. *Wound Rep Regen* **7**: 172–8

Steed DL (1995) Clinical evaluation of recombinant human platelet-derived growth factor for the treatment of lower extremity diabetic ulcers. Diabetic Ulcer Study Group. *J Vasc Surg* **21**: 71–8

Steed DL, Goslen JB, Holloway GA, Malone JM, Bunt TJ, Webster MW (1992) Randomized prospective double-blind trial in healing chronic diabetic foot ulcers. CT-102 activated platelet supernatant, topical versus placebo. *Diabetes Care* **15**: 1598–604

Steffensen B, Hakkinen L, Larjava H (2001) Proteolytic events of wound-healing — coordinated interactions among matrix metalloproteinases (MMPs), integrins, and extracellular matrix molecules. *Crit Rev Oral Biol Med* **12**: 373–98

Streit M, Braathen LR (2000) Apligraf — a living human skin equivalent for the treatment of chronic wounds. *Int J Artif Organs* **23**: 831–3

Tarlton JF, Bailey AJ, Crawford E, Jones D, Moore K, Harding KD (1999) Rognostic value of markers of collagen remodeling in venous ulcers. *Wound Repair Regen* **7**: 347–55

Thomas A, Harding KG, Moore K (2000) Alginates from wound dressings activate human macrophages to secrete tumour necrosis factor-alpha. *Biomaterials* **21**: 1797–802

Trengove N, Stacey MC, McGechie DF, Stingemore NF, Mata S (1996). Qualitative bacteriology and leg ulcer healing. *J Wound Care* **5**: 277–80

Trengove NJ, Stacey MC, MacAuley S *et al* (1999) Analysis of the acute and chronic wound environments: the role of proteases and their inhibitors. *Wound Rep Regen* **7**(6): 442–52

Valencia IC, Falabella AF, Eaglstein WH (2000) Skin grafting. *Dermatol Clin* **18**: 521–32

Vin F, Teot L, Meaume S (2002) The healing properties of Promogran in venous leg ulcers. *J Wound Care* **11**: 335–41

West DC, Kumar S (1989) The effect of hyaluronate and its oligosaccharides on endothelial cell proliferation and monolayer integrity. *Exp Cell Res* **183**: 179–96

White RJ (2003) An historical overview of the use of silver in wound management. In: White RJ, ed. *The Silver Book*. Quay Books, MA Healthcare Limited, Dinton, Salisbury: 59–68

Winter G D (1962) Formation of the scab and the rate of epithelisation of superficial wounds in the skin of the young domestic pig. *Nature* **193**: 293–94

Wright TE, Hill DP, Ko F *et al* (2000) The effect of TGF-beta2 in various vehicles on incisional wound healing. *Int J Surg Investig* **2**: 133–43

Xia YP, Zhao Y, Marcus J *et al* (1999) Effects of keratinocyte growth factor-2 (KGF-2) on wound healing in an ischaemia-impaired rabbit ear model and on scar formation. *J Pathol* **188**: 431–8

Yager DR, Chen SM, Ward SI (1997) Ability of chronic wound fluids to degrade peptide growth factors is associated with increased levels of elastase activity and diminished levels of proteinase inhibitors. *Wound Rep Regen* **5**: 23–32

10

Barriers to the implementation of clinical guidelines

Michael Clark

Clinical guidelines in wound care have recently been formulated at the national and international level, reflecting a shift from locally derived guidelines common during the 1990s. There remains considerable uncertainty regarding the extent of implementation and monitoring of these new guidelines. This chapter presents the results of a survey of members of the Tissue Viability Society that sought their views upon the guidelines in place within their workplace — how were these guidelines developed? was the impact of guidelines monitored? and how, and finally, what barriers limited their full implementation? Of the 1500 members, 476 returned completed questionnaires (34.0% response rate). Most (n=422, 88.4%) worked within environments that implemented clinical guidelines in some aspect of wound care, with guidance upon pressure ulcer prevention being most commonly reported (n=351). The use of national guidelines (either in their original format or locally modified to reflect local circumstances) was relatively common — reported by 307 of the 476 respondents. Few reported that guidelines were fully implemented (n=77; 18.3%) with lack of resources, lack of awareness of the content of the guidelines and, when aware, lack of acceptance of their recommendations being the most commonly cited reasons for the failure to implement. However, it should be noted that only 34.0% of the surveyed population responded — this may question how far the results can be considered to reflect the current status of guideline implementation in the UK given the unreported views of 66% of all those surveyed.

Clinical guidelines have been defined as 'systematically developed statements to assist practitioner and patient decisions about appropriate health care for specific clinical circumstances' (Effective Health Care, 1994). It is undisputed that the implementation of valid, reliable guidelines can positively affect both the processes and outcomes of health care (Effective Health Care, 1994). However, there remains considerable debate regarding the 'best' approach to their development, implementation and monitoring (Clark, 1999). For example ,should a wound care guideline be developed at an international, national or local level? If developed nationally how can the implementation of the guideline at a local level be best achieved? Not least among the questions that surround the evaluation of guideline use is how are practitioners and health-care managers to evaluate the impact of guideline implementation? National and international guidelines in wound care are relatively common; within pressure ulcer prevention and treatment alone at least twelve national and European level guidelines exist. In the UK, this profusion of national guidelines is well illustrated by the concurrent availability of the National Institute for Clinical Excellence (NICE) pressure ulcer guidelines (NICE, 2001), the Clinical Resource Efficiency Support Team guideline in Northern Ireland (Clinical Resource Efficiency Spport Team, 1998) and the European Pressure Ulcer Advisory Panel's (EPUAP) guidelines on prevention and treatment (EPUAP, 1998; 1999) among others.

National guidelines on pressure ulceration are a relatively recent phenomenon in the UK with the oldest dating back to 1998. Ten years ago the emphasis was firmly placed upon the development of local initiatives (King's Fund Centre, 1989). Despite such emphasis, it was considered by the National Audit Office (NAO) (Booth, 1992) that relatively few local pressure ulcer guidelines existed. To identify whether local guidelines were more common than was believed by the NAO, Watts and Clark (Panel for the Prediction and Prevention of Pressure Ulcers in Adults, 1992) reported a national survey of the number and content of pressure ulcer prevention policies implemented within NHS trusts, health authorities and individual hospitals. This postal survey sent out 397 questionnaires with 325 returned (response rate 81.8%). From the respondents, 138 had locally developed pressure ulcer prevention guidelines with a further forty-five stated to be in development at the time of the survey. In 1993, it appeared that pressure ulcer guidelines were already relatively commonplace in UK health care. Of the guidelines reported to Watts and Clark, eighty-six were made available for review and of these the majority (*n*=50; 58.3%) had been compiled by multidisciplinary groups, although the guideline contents were often solely directed towards nursing practices.

In 1998, the EPUAP guideline on pressure ulcer prevention was issued and to explore its likely impact, a second postal questionnaire was undertaken in the summer of 1998 (Grey and Clark, unpublished data, 1998). In this survey of 150 UK tissue viability specialist nurses, responses were received from 34.6% (*n*=52). Most respondents followed a pressure ulcer prevention guideline (*n*=45; 86.5%) with thirty-nine of these being locally derived. Where national guidelines were in place; five (working in Scotland) implemented nationally derived guidelines in Scotland while a single respondent implemented the United States Agency for Health Care Policy and Research pressure ulcer guidelines (Panel for the Prediction and Prevention of Pressure Ulcers in Adults, 1992). From this, albeit limited response from the nurses surveyed, locally derived guidelines were in common use in the late 1990s.

While these surveys of the use of locally and nationally derived pressure ulcer guidelines provide insights into the number and origin of guidelines in place in the UK during the 1990s they provide little information about the extent of guideline implementation, nor do they identify the barriers, if any, to full guideline implementation. Watts and Clark (1993) inferred that the implementation of the guidelines reported in their survey may have been limited. This conclusion was drawn from four observations — only two guidelines gave information upon the size of the local problem of pressure ulceration, in 75% of guidelines there was no assistance provided to help staff obtain further copies, only 49% included any references within their guideline and, finally, only 35% identified staff training needs. These indirect, and perhaps weak, indicators of guideline implementation are the only information regarding the extent of pressure ulcer guideline implementation in the UK during the last decade.

To explore current trends in wound care guideline development, implementation and monitoring a postal questionnaire was administered to all members of the Tissue Viability Society during the summer of 2002. The present report summarises the responses of the membership of the Tissue Viability Society while raising issues related to the interpretation of relatively low questionnaire response rates.

Methods

A questionnaire was developed, consisting of six questions covering:

⌘ The respondent's main role in their workplace.
⌘ The aspects of wound care delivery that were covered by clinical guidelines.
⌘ How were the guidelines developed?
⌘ How was the impact of the guidelines monitored?
⌘ What barriers existed (if any) to achieving the full implementation of the guidelines?
⌘ How could the Tissue Viability Society best help its members to develop and implement clinical guidelines?

This questionnaire was published in the *Journal of Tissue Viability* to raise awareness of its subsequent circulation to members (Anonymous, 2002). Following publication the questionnaire was posted to 1500 members of the Tissue Viability Society during the summer of 2002. Each member received the questionnaire and a pre-paid envelope facilitating its return to the Business Office of the Tissue Viability Society. All questionnaires were to be completed anonymously and no identification of the respondent was possible from the returned form.

Results

Four hundred and seventy-six completed questionnaires were returned to the Tissue Viability Society office; a response rate of 34.0%. Most of the questionnaires had been completed by nurses (n=183; 38.4%), with a further 167 (35.1%) returned by clinical nurse specialists in tissue viability. No other single professional group returned more than forty questionnaires (*Table 10.1*).

The majority of respondents stated that they worked within an environment which implemented clinical guidelines in some aspect of wound care (n=422; 88.4%). The fifty-five respondents who reported no guideline use provided the foremost reason they had not adopted guidelines (*Table 10.2*). For many (n=26; 47.3%) clinical guidelines were inappropriate (for example, those in commerce and research) while a further thirteen noted that guidelines were being prepared but had not yet been implemented. Seven respondents noted a variety of reasons why guidelines were not implemented ranging from lack of relevant guidelines (*n*=3; paediatric palliative care, seating, one unspecified), guidelines in place but not available in their department (*n*=1), a lack of a local 'expert' to promote guidelines (*n*=2) and, finally, to the presence of large numbers of temporary staff (part-time, agency or bank nurses) (*n*=1).

Where guidelines were followed; the most commonly reported guideline topic was pressure ulcer prevention (*n*=351; *Figure 10.1*). Many respondents noted that multiple topics were covered by guidelines, hence the numbers shown in *Figure 10.1* exceed the total number of respondents. Twenty further clinical topics were also reported to be covered by guidelines by some respondents (*Table 10.3*), with guidelines covering the management of diabetic foot ulcers being most frequently reported (*n*=15 respondents). Five clinical guidelines addressed the use of larval

Table 10.1: Professional roles of the Tissue Viability Society members who returned completed questionnaires

Role	Number of respondents
Nursing	183
Clinical nurse specialist tissue viability	167
Profession allied to medicine	36
Education	21
Nurse specialist (unspecified)	16
Management	15
Research	13
Medicine	10
Commerce	10
Other (pharmacy, podiatry, practice development, district nursing community practice teacher)	4
Not reported	1
Total	**476**

Table 10.2: Were clinical guidelines covering some aspect of wound management followed by the respondents?

Were clinical guidelines followed?	Number of respondents
Yes	422
No	55
Why were guidelines not in use	
Inappropriate to workplace	26
In development but not yet implemented	13
Other reason	7
No response	5
No interest	3
Guidelines not required	1

therapy with four guidelines tackling use of negative pressure therapies.

It was possible that the guidelines that were implemented could have been developed at an international, national or local level. Respondents were asked to identify the source of their guidelines – as many followed several guidelines, frequently respondents selected more than one 'level' of guideline development. The highest level of guideline development (for example, international then national then local based on national guidelines) identified by each respondent is shown in *Figure 10.2*. Sixty-six (13.8%) respondents followed international guidelines while a higher number (*n*=107; 22.5%) adopted nationally derived guidelines. However, the single largest group had adapted national guidelines to better reflect their local circumstances (*n*=200; 42.0%).

Table 10.3: Additional clinical topics reported to be addressed using clinical guidelines

Topic	Number of respondents
Management of diabetic foot ulcers	15
Larval therapy	5
Negative pressure therapy	4
Management of arterial leg ulcers	4
Management of 'all leg ulcers'	3
'General wound care'	2
Reactions to radiotherapy	2
Sharp debridement, traumatic wounds, nutrition, infection control, lymphoedema management, removal of drains, skin barrier creams, surgical wounds, 'care pathways', skin protection, mattresses, cushions, measurement of interface pressure	All of these were noted by single respondents

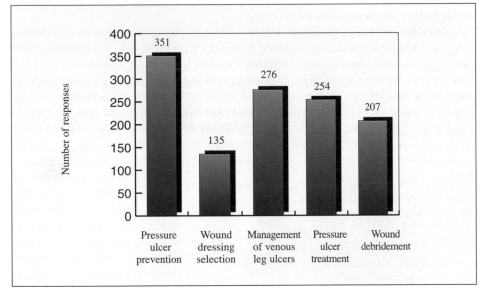

Figure 10.1: Clinical topics reported to be covered by clinical guidelines

Among those who worked with clinical guidelines, most monitored the success of their guidelines (*n*=358; 75.2%); however, fifty-six did not monitor guidelines and seven did not answer this question. *Figure 10.3* illustrates the key methods used to monitor the impact of guidelines with outcome audits measuring prevalence or incidence of wounds being the most commonly reported technique (*n*=240; respondents made multiple responses to this question hence the total responses shown in *Figure 10.3* exceeds the number of respondents). Other forms of auditing the successful implementation of guidelines were reported (twelve methods each mentioned by a single respondent). These included monitoring of complaints, discussion within link nurse groups and during study days, audits of dressing use and measurement of healing rates.

Of the 421 respondents who followed clinical guide-lines, seventy- seven (18.3%) considered their guideline(s) to be fully implemented while thirty-nine failed to answer this question. Among the 305 who considered imple-mentation was incomplete the single most commonly reported barrier was lack of resources (*n*=151, *Table 10.4*).

Table 10.4: Reported barriers to full guideline implementation

Barrier	*n*
Lack of resources	151
Lack of awareness of guideline content	144
Lack of acceptance of guideline recommendations	65
Uncertain how to monitor the guideline	62
Failure of guideline to identify clearly best practice	42
Evidence base too weak to support recommendations	27
Guideline topic not considered important	26
Guideline impractical within care setting	19
Significant concerns overlooked within guideline	18

Respondents also noted several other barriers, including; lack of managerial acceptance of the guideline (n=3), lack of staff training and lack of staff interest (*n*=2 in both cases), low staff levels (*n*=2) and changes in the organization of community care (*n*=1).

The final question posed to Tissue Viability Society members considered whether, and how, the Society should best help with guideline development and implementation. Most Tissue Viability Society members considered that the Society did have a role to play in assisting the most effective use of guidelines (*n*=410 of the 421 who followed guidelines; 97.4%), with six failing to answer this question. Only five considered that the Society had no role to play in guideline introduction and monitoring. *Figure 10.4* shows the major activities that the Tissue Viability Society should consider undertaking (the number of responses exceeds the 421 who followed guideline use). The most prevalent opinion was that the Tissue Viability Society should promote awareness of guide-lines and their content (*n*=325). Many other suggestions were offered regarding the potential role of the Tissue Viability Society; of these, only one was reported by more than a single respondent — two believed the Tissue Viability Society should exert greater pressure upon the Department of Health to consider tissue viability as a 'high priority' in health care.

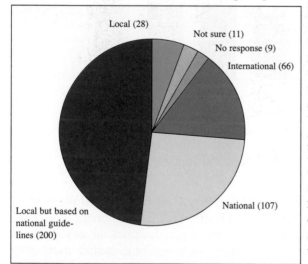

Figure 10.2: Level of development of reported wound care guidelines. This figure shows the highest level of development reported by respondents — for example, an individual may pursue three guidelines — derived at the local, national or international levels — the figure would represent this individual at the international level

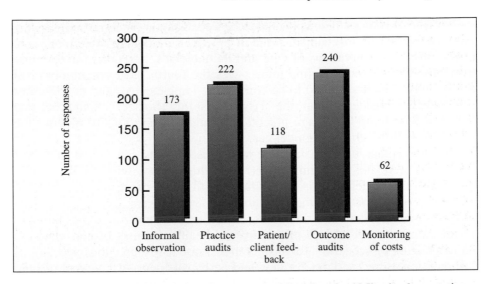

Figure 10.3: Methods used to monitor the success or otherwise of guideline implementation

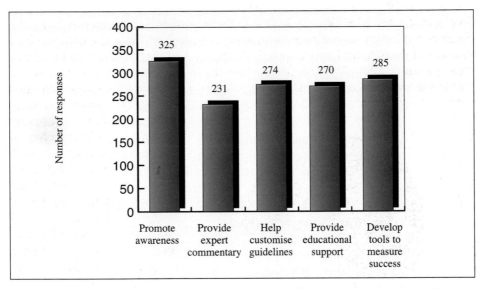

Figure 10.4: Methods through which the Tissue Viability Society could enhance its role in guideline development, implementation and monitoring

Conclusions

This survey of the members of the Tissue Viability Society has identified a major shift in the use of clinical practice guidelines in wound care over the last five years — where previously guidelines, although commonplace, were developed at a local level, it would now appear that national and international guidelines have begun to play a greater role in shaping wound care.

Monitoring of the impact of guidelines was also commonly reported in the present survey with 75.2% of all those who followed guidelines monitoring their effect. However, there appeared to be a focus upon outcome audits as the primary monitoring mechanism – and in 173 cases guidelines were monitored using informal observations of care and its outcomes. A reported uncertainty over how to monitor guideline impact was the fourth most commonly cited reason why guidelines failed to be completely implemented, and in 285 cases respondents considered that the Tissue Viability Society should become involved in helping healthcare practitioners and organisations to monitor the impact of their wound care guidelines.

It was perhaps unsurprising that many respondents considered that their guidelines were not fully implemented. In this survey, only 18.3% ($n=77$) reported full guideline implementation, with lack of resources, lack of awareness of the content of the guidelines and, when aware, lack of acceptance of their recommendations being the three key reasons why guidelines failed to be fully implemented. A lack of resources in health care may be considered to be an unchanging scenario – for any given increase in resource the expectations of practitioners and patients for new and perhaps expensive interventions are likely to increase. However, it is relevant to consider how guideline content can best be introduced to staff while simultaneously overcoming any barriers to the acceptance of their recommendations – this is one area where the Tissue Viability Society may help advance the use of guidelines in wound care. Given the Society's well established educational events and national conferences, it would appear to be possible to include sessions on guidelines and their content during such gatherings.

While it is tempting to consider that the views of the 476 respondents well reflect the overall extent of guideline development in the UK, the respondents reflected a minority of all those issued with the questionnaire. The views and experiences of the silent majority (66.0%) of all those surveyed may reflect different views on wound care guidelines in the UK. This uncertainty regarding how representative the views of the respondents actually were must limit the conclusions of the survey — perhaps those who responded had particularly strong views on guidelines with either positive or negative experiences?

Key points

⌘ Wound care guidelines and, in particular, pressure ulcer clinical guidelines are relatively common across UK healthcare. There has been a shift over the past few years from these guidelines being locally developed towards the current guidelines being locally adapted versions of national and international guidelines.

⌘ Lack of resources plays a major role in limiting the implementation of clinical guidelines, as does lack of awareness of the guideline and lack of acceptance of guideline recommendations.

⌘ There remains little information regarding the clinical outcomes obtained, and financial costs incurred, when implementing wound care guidelines.

References

Anonymous (2002) Use of guidelines in tissue viability. *J Tissue Viability* **12**(3): 122–3

Booth B (1992) Pressing problem. *Nurs Times* **88**(31): 19

Clark M (1999) Developing guidelines for pressure ulcer prevention and management. *J Wound Care* **8**(7): 357–9

Clinical Resource Efficiency Support Team (1998) *Guidelines for the Prevention and Management of Pressure Sores. Recommendations for Practice*. Clinical Resource Efficiency Support Team, Belfast

Effective Health Care (1994) *Implementing Clinical Practice Guidelines. Can guidelines be used to improve clinical practice?* University of Leeds, Leeds

European Pressure Ulcer Advisory Panel (1998) Pressure ulcer prevention guidelines. *Br J Nurs* **7**(15): 888–9

European Pressure Ulcer Advisory Panel (1999) Guidelines on treatment of pressure ulcers. *EPUAP Review* **1**(2): 31–3

King's Fund Centre (1989) The prevention and management of pressure sores within health districts: A document produced by the working party of the pressure sore study group at the King's Fund Centre for Health Services Development. King's Fund Centre, London

National Institute for Clinical Excellence (2001) *Pressure Ulcer Risk Management and Prevention (Inherited Guideline B)*. NICE, London

Panel for the Prediction and Prevention of Pressure Ulcers in Adults (1992) Pressure Ulcers in Adults: Prediction and Prevention. Clinical practice guideline Number 3. Rockville, MD: Agency for Health Care Policy and Research, Public Health Service, Department of Health and Human Services, US

Watts S, Clark M (1993) *Pressure sore prevention: a review of policy documents. Final Report to the Department of Health*. University of Surrey, Guildford

Index